The Lotus Files

© 2012

Larissa C Walters

For Brenda...

ACKNOWLEDGMENTS

There are so many people to thank as I would have never completed this memoir on my own. To each and every person who encouraged me over the past two years, I'm still standing because of you. The little gems you deposited in my spirit along the way have made me richer than any monetary amount could.

A Special Thank You to:
My Father, Grandma Sarah, Aunt Jackie, and Kelly for loving Brenda as much as I did in your own ways. The love you gave her was also given to me.

Courtney Savoy of A-List Graphics, for being such a Dear Friend and the Book Cover Designer.

Photographer Extraordinaire, Paul "P.A." Greene for my Author Images.

Dear Family Friend Keith Ross, who planted the original seed that my blog was actually my book.

My personal Editors: Andre Dubose, Rolanda Prophete, Eboni Thomas, Marche Taylor, Amanda Bevilacqua, Robert Snowden, Patricia Spady-Dubose, and Meagan Brown. Thank you for confirming that I had a responsibility to share my story.

CONTENTS

1. PROLOGUE-YOU ARE NOT ALONE (6/1/11)

This book is my personal journey of the toughest year of my life. What makes this year so significant is that sadly, this is a year that nearly every human being will face at some point in his or her life. It's the first year after a tragic loss of a dear loved one. I've learned that there is no preparation for that year. Whether you had time before the loved one crossed over or they were taken in the blink of an eye without warning, the pain is the same. The questions, the hurt, the despair, and the loneliness are the same. The only difference is the process. As I went through my process, I learned the hard way that not everyone would understand what I was going through nor did they have to. It wasn't their journey therefore their vantage point was going to be different. However, I did find that as much as I felt alone and lonely (there is a difference), I was finding this unspoken camaraderie with those who had walked this path before me as well as with those who started on the path after me.

I started a blog shortly after I received news that my mother's nine-year on and off battle with breast cancer was coming to an end. It started out as a way for me to vent about my confusion, fear, rage and frustrations as a means to not keep them pent up. I thought that perhaps I'd be able to help someone else along the way but I must admit that my intentions in the beginning were more of a selfish nature. I simply needed a sounding board for the

___

unexplainable roller coaster of emotions I was going through.

What developed over the following year as I continued to chronicle my experiences turned into the most beautiful and humbling evolution I could have ever imagined. The feedback I received was consistently positive. Friends, family, and complete strangers would let me know how the blog was helping them cope with their process or even showing them how to be there for a loved one who was knee deep in the process. The overwhelming message that I kept getting was that I wasn't alone in my feelings. While no one will ever know the major and minor nuances of my journey, there were some consistent themes that assured me that although I couldn't see the light at the end of the tunnel, someone had been in my space before and I'd eventually be in a better place emotionally, spiritually, and mentally.

I read different books on grieving and the one thing I didn't find was a personal account of the first year after losing a loved one. This is notoriously the worst year as it contains all of the "first" milestones without them. Holidays, birthdays, anniversaries, good news, bad news, and no news, all hold different meaning now. And when you really get caught up in your emotions, you realize that these milestones represent the rest of your "new" life.

I decided that I would share my journey and convert the blog into a book so that maybe someone could have a slightly easier way than I did. Knowing that in the midst of their grieving, they are not alone even when they feel like they are. It's my mission to ensure that no one else has that moment of doubt because as I have learned, there is strength in numbers.

I cried, screamed, broke things, laughed, and surprised myself on this journey. I've unlocked pieces of myself that I didn't know existed. I found courage that I never knew I had and I'm a stronger person for it. My hope is that as you walk on this path with me, you feel all of the emotions, triumphs, and valleys that I did and while doing so, make a connection. Whether it is to love someone going through this journey a little harder, or to love yourself harder because sometimes you have to do that too. You're not crazy. You've been chosen to be strong without the person who once gave you strength. The reason why you were chosen is because you're already strong enough. Finding that strength within, while grieving, is the ultimate challenge.

I'm sharing my experience with you to remind you that you will make it to the other side of the pain, because I did. Not to ever say that it goes away because it doesn't. I still have my good and horrible days. But how you react to and embrace the pain will get easier, one day at a time.

I know without doubt or confusion that in the darkest part of your grief, one day at a time is all you have. You are not alone.

2. FIRST IN A LONG JOURNEY (1/29/10)

On January 5th 2010, I received news that would permanently change my life. I was informed that My Best Friend, My Mentor, My Hero, My Mother's nine year battle with Breast Cancer was coming to an end sooner than any of us could have predicted as the cancer spread to her brain. The doctor looked me right in the eyes and told me frankly and sympathetically that my mother had 3-6 months, maybe longer to live. Within a week and a half that timeline dropped to "weeks to months".

To some, I would be considered lucky because I still have time to spend and create memories. But to walk in my shoes these last couple of weeks, I feel anything but lucky. I'm going through the first of two grieving processes that others who have lost a loved one go through once. I'm grieving the inevitable loss of my mother while watching the strongest, proudest woman I know rapidly decline physically. Someone who could slowly walk on her own on the 5th of January, can now only get around in a wheelchair because her motor skills are deteriorating. And the only reason that I will get through this initial grieving process is because...she'll be gone. Let the second grieving process begin. Lucky me.

Although coined the strong one amongst family and friends, I'm not ready for this and everyday is a new set of emotions to work through. My hope is that through writing my feelings down, I can help myself and ultimately help someone else going through a similar situation. I know I'm not alone and I have a support system that loves me. But it's a lot easier to relate to someone who's been there.

I named this blog (and now book) The Lotus Files because the Lotus flower journeys through dark, and murky waters to bloom into a beautiful flower on top of that water. That's what I believe is happening to my mother and I. Hopefully, I can help someone else out along the way.

3. TODAY WAS A GOOD DAY *(1/31/10)*

The biggest struggle for me so far has been coping with the contrast between the poker face I put on when I'm with my mom and dealing with the reality of how I feel when not in her presence. It's almost schizophrenic. I was scheduled to fly home Friday evening and had to switch my flight to Saturday morning because I couldn't get it together emotionally. This past week was by far the worst at this juncture for me. I can count one day where I was "okay". Other than that, it was wise to stay out of my way because I was pissed at the world and my alter ego Laquita was on a warpath. I've taken up yoga to give myself some balance but it's still a process.

If you're wondering why I'm subjecting myself to this Jekyll and Hyde persona, it's simply because with the time we have left, mom deserves to see nothing but happiness and smiles so I choose to check all negativity and sadness at the door when I come home. Of course she's my mother and can sense my hurt but I know it means a lot to her to see my smiling face rather than a sad one.

I was pleasantly surprised when I came home today to see that her speech had improved significantly. It was actually almost back to normal. Since the cancer progressed, her speech had become slurred to the point where I had to look at her lips to understand her. I walked in her room to see the BIG smile I know and love and was able to have a normal conversation.

I'm amazed by the peace she has. My mother is very passionate and emotional and has never had an issue displaying how she feels over the years. Since the fateful appointment where the doctor told her the prognosis she has yet to cry about it. A part of me is still waiting for her to hit the wall, but my spirit knows that somehow she's accepted the inevitable. I'm just not there yet, but I'm working on it.

We laughed and joked today like we always do. She had a visitor, and we wrapped the day up by doing some online shopping at Tiffany's (the Blue Box always helps). The doctors said that she would improve for a little while after her radiation was over so I'm definitely enjoying this time and don't feel as robbed as I did on my last visit when her decline happened within a week and half. We'll put this day in the books as a good one and I'll sleep a little easier tonight.

4. SOMEONE'S SHOWING OFF *(2/1/10)*

Today was pretty quiet. Mom sleeps a lot now and today it rubbed off on me. We woke up in time to watch The Grammys and between that and the Twitter updates; I got some much-needed laughs. Mom got a little choked up during Mary J Blige's rendition of "Like a Bridge" and reiterated that that's the song she wants me to sing at her Home Going Celebration. This request always weird's me out, so I simply nodded knowing damn well that I won't be able to squeak a note because I'll be too choked up. Moving on....

The ray of sunshine today was seeing her improvement with her balance and mobility. She still needs the wheelchair but I pretty much just stood by and watched her make her way from the bed to the wheelchair. She started showing off and did a little dance while standing up that we do when we're playing around. It made us both laugh. I'm definitely enjoying this time and staying in the moment though I'd be lying if I said that the fear of her decline isn't in the back of my head. The Radiologist said that her function would improve after the radiation is done so this period of improvement is bittersweet because it's only supposed to be temporary.

I am grateful though. I was so deflated after I left last weekend because I didn't have any warning about how quickly she lost function. I feel like I've been given a second chance to mentally prepare myself for what's next. Because of that, I'm assured that I'm only given what I can bear. Another good day in the books for us!

5. THE TOUGH PART *(2/2/10)*

This is my last night home before heading back to Baltimore. My parents live in Albany, NY so that makes leaving all the more difficult because mom's not around the corner. It's an hour plane ride and a 5.5 hour drive so needless to say my constant traveling as of late is taxing and doesn't help my concerns for her when I'm not here. I'll take this good weekend with me though. No matter what happens next, I was given the opportunity to have my mother with me, the way I know her, when I didn't know if I'd have that chance again. I had her smile, her laugh, her silliness, and her GENUINE, UNCONDITIONAL love for me. I see it every time she looks at me...so proud even though I haven't done half of the things I want to do for her or accomplished half of the things I want to accomplish yet. Through everything she's my biggest fan. No judgment in her eyes...only support.

I am who I am because of her and I'm not half the fighter or spirit she is. She gives me something to aim for. We had a heart to heart tonight. I wrote down several questions that I wanted her to answer via video camera. At first, understandingly, she didn't want to do it but she decided recently that she would. She answered some of my questions for me. I asked her if she was scared and if so what was she scared of...she told me. She told me she was most afraid of what she would be missing, like seeing me get married, having children and that it wasn't fair. At that point we both choked up. She also told me she was afraid of not being here for me. It's not that she doesn't believe that I'll be okay but because she knows how heavily I rely on her for guidance. She told me that I need to begin to look within and trust myself because she will always be in my heart and whatever answers I need in life will be there. I asked her about my spiritual gifts and a few other things that I needed just for me and shall remain between us.

My mother's life wasn't easy but she took all of the negativity and flipped it into love and placed it in me. So many people take life's blows and never share their stories and testimonies. She decided at an early age that I would be the exception and she would break the cycle with me. For that, I'm grateful.

I'm amazed at how many people have come out of the woodwork because my mother touched them over the years. People who she hasn't seen or heard from since 1983 when my dad was in the Air Force stationed in Florida, have been calling because they got word about her condition, and just wanted to remind her of how she blessed them. With one of these calls I learned that she was in the delivery room with an old friend as she was giving birth to her daughter. My eyes got so big while listening to the story as I imagined my mother helping this lady give birth! Easy to turn green, I literally passed out once watching a colonoscopy in an operating room! I can laugh at myself because I know I'm pitiful! What a great legacy Brenda has! If I can accomplish half of the

things she has in 55 years with the odds against her, my
prayer will be answered!

6. BLAH... *(2/3/10)*

I'm back in Baltimore and leaving mom wasn't as bad as the last time. I kept myself busy today as to not worry and I'm okay. I'll be back with her in a week for a big doctor's appointment, so all I can do now is wait in anticipation. My dad likened it to patching up and stocking a battered boat the best you can, setting it out to sea, and hoping for the best. I know my mother is stubborn and has no intentions of leaving here until she's good and ready so I believe that boat will be afloat for longer than we think and that's completely fine with me.

7. I'M AN OC *(2/4/10)*

As an Only Child (OC), this walk poses some unique
challenges. It's always been just my mom, my dad, and
me. Because my dad was in the Air Force when I was
child we were always our own little unit. We never lived
close to extended family so my bond with my parents is a
little different than most. My mother and I definitely had
tough times when I was growing up as any
teenager/parent relationship goes. I recall times when
she would work my LAST NERVE because she was so
damn strict! My best friend growing up and I were SO
sheltered. I can look back on it and laugh now but it
sucked going through it. It wasn't until my
Sophomore/Junior year in college that our relationship
changed to what it is today but we still had some bumps
and bruises along the way.

I share all this to illustrate the bond my mother and I
have. It's always been JUST me! All of the hopes and
dreams parents have for their children to do better than
them fell on me. I didn't have any siblings to share
growing pains with back then and I don't have any
siblings to share them with now. Perhaps a sibling would
know exactly how I feel, and how I worry. Perhaps a
sibling would understand exactly why I can't fall asleep
until 3 or 4 in the morning. Perhaps a sibling could look
me in the eyes and tell me genuinely that they know
exactly where I'm at emotionally. Perhaps a sibling could
share the pressure, but I'm an OC. So I bear these feelings

and emotions solely. It's a blessing and a curse.

My mom is one of the most selfless people I know. However, in that selflessness, I never had to share her. She was and is all mine. We're Best Friends because of it. I never had to compete with someone else for her Love because I always had all of it. She was able to pour all of herself into me and me only. Over the years, I acquired the nickname BJ or Brenda Jr. I fought it at first as most youngsters do but I hold the banner up with pride now. I'm both my mother's daughter and my father's son, and I honestly wouldn't have it any other way.

8. GROWING PAINS *(2/7/10)*

So much for a full week without a meltdown. And to think that I was doing so well! Although writing is helping me, at the same time, with all the help in the world, I'm still not the light-spirited person I'm known to be since January 5th. Frankly, I don't feel that I have to be and anyone who feels that I've changed over this past month is right. I have changed. I'm in the middle of an unwarranted metamorphosis and every day is different. Everyday even with its little joys and moments still sucks because I ultimately know what's waiting for me at the end of this journey.

I've been trying to keep my deep seeded anger in check but it's not working. My tolerance level is nil to none. I don't have it in me to be the person I was before 1:30pm on January 5th and I don't know when I will. I'd like to think that over time I'll be that individual again, but that individual had her Best Friend. The "New" me won't. I'd like to think that I'll be better because of this but the light at the end of the tunnel is currently non-existent. With that being said, is it fair to subject those who are used to seeing me happy and full of advice to my negative tirades? On the other hand, is it fair for them to expect me to be the same and in turn not adjust their interaction with me?

I don't feel that I'm difficult to understand nor do I feel that I require more than what I offer to those close to me.

I am finding myself lost in between and that leaves
me frustrated. I don't think that I'm too good or too strong
to talk about my feelings and anger. However, I release
them in my own time. Not everyone gets that. Forcing me
to feel better by "making" me talk or subjecting me to
unwarranted humor are not the routes. At my wits end,
cue in my evil Gemini twin "Laquita".

My phone was the sacrificial lamb today. In a fit of rage, it
was thrown across the living room and subsequently
broken leaving the face cracked and with no picture.
Fortunately, my insurance plan will have me with a new
phone by Tuesday. I'm learning along the way to deal with
this and as much as I try to control my uncontrollable
feelings, sometimes they get the best of me. I heard a
quote today that said "Screw the results, relish the
process". I'm trying, but why is it that I feel better
relishing it by myself?

9. WHAT A WEEK! IS IT OVER YET? *(2/12/10)*

What a week! I came to Albany on Tuesday to avoid the "Snowpacalypse" in Maryland and it wasn't without drama. I can look back on it and laugh now so I'll share because I don't want to be a complete Debbie Downer as I share my story. Laughing at myself has never been an issue and there's always an occasion for some reason!

So Monday night, my parents booked my flight out on Tuesday so I could beat the snowstorm in order to attend my mother's "really important" doctor's appointment on Thursday. Mind you I still had the broken phone from throwing it across the room over the weekend. So Tuesday morning I woke up ready to get the day started. I made arrangements at 10am for a taxi to pick me up by 12:15 for my 2:20 flight and got ready. At 12:15, no cab, so I Instant Messaged my boyfriend on my computer to call the cab company because I couldn't call out on my broken phone. They were surprised the cab hadn't come and assured us it was on its way. At 12:30 I got nervous and reluctantly grabbed my shovel to dig my car out of the 24+ inches of snow "just in case" I had to drive myself to the airport.

I walked out the door with shovel in hand and a little cockiness because I'm from Rochester NY aka "The ROC". All of that snow was not foreign to me. I totally had it under control (or so I thought). So my freshly straightened hair and I began to shovel. The terms:

comedic tragedy, hot mess, and ultimate failure do not BEGIN to describe my 5'3, 120 pound stature trying to shovel all that damn snow! 20+ inches to be exact! Adding insult to injury, my neighbors watched me scuffle for about 40 minutes before they offered their assistance. Meanwhile, still NO cab! The dispatcher even called me to let me know the cab was outside my door, except it was on the North side of the Avenue and not the South where I live.

Annnnd we're shoveling! We FINALLY dug my car out at 1:30. I threw my luggage in the car and attempted to high tail it to the airport where my flight was taking off at 2:20. Of course the roads were a nightmare and I couldn't even leave stank ass Baltimore because the main arteries to get out of downtown were all backed up. Exasperated, at 1:50 I called my mother and told her to cancel the flight because I clearly was not going to make it on time.

At that point, I was still wearing my sopping wet socks and Timberlands from shoveling and decided that I'd have to drive to Albany ASAP. But before I did anything else, I decided to go home to at least change my wet socks. En route home, my little Honda Accord Coupe got stuck in the snow around the corner from my house. Thank the Lord for two Good Samaritans who helped me make it through that travesty! One was an older lady who steered my car while we pushed it (and if she was crazy, could have drove off once we freed it). The other was a gentleman who busted his ass and fell face first trying to help me push my car out of the snow. Although I wanted to laugh so badly (after I established he was okay) while helping him up, I found a way to hold it in.

I finally got on the road and it was just starting to snow again but I beat out the storm once I hit the Scranton PA area. All in all, my would be hour flight turned into a 6.5 hour drive not counting the melee I went through to get out of the city to beat the storm all thanks to the trifling taxi company. Are you laughing yet?! And just for kicks and giggles, the taxi company called me at 1:35 to let me know they made it to my house. It took everything in me to keep Laquita from making another appearance on that poor dispatcher!

I made it home around 10pm and was met with multiple jokes about my hair that was no longer freshly straightened and actually looked like I went to Sideshow Bob from the Simpsons' hairstylist instead since I sweat my hair out shoveling about 8 hours prior. It was good to see that mom still had her sense of humor!

I went through all of that so I could obviously be home with my mom but mostly so I could make this "really important" doctor's appointment on Thursday. Well today's Thursday and the appointment wound up not being that important. This fool of a doctor "assessed" my mother and asked us if we had any questions. Um, yeah fool, how about those "alternative methods" you were supposed to be "researching"?! Of course he said he didn't find anything, and we were left with "Letting Go & Letting God".

The only reason why I'm handling this well is because my mother's improvement is markedly better.
She gets around with her walker now and doesn't even need the wheelchair. Her speech is better and her spirits are surprisingly good! Not too bad for a woman who couldn't walk on her own a week ago. I told y'all she was a fighter! So we'll see what the near future holds but mom is planning a cruise next month and knowing her she has no intentions of wasting her money. I truly love that woman!

10. GO GIRL, IT'S YOUR BIRTHDAY *(2/13/10)*

My Aunt who I affectionately refer to as "Aunteee" and
Uncle are visiting my parents from Warner Robins
Georgia this week. They bring great comic relief and a
nice change of pace. Aunteee always keeps it real and
holds no punches. We've been estranged for most of my
life but her and my mother (sisters) have mended their
relationship over the last couple of years and I have to
admit that it's nice to have them around. Today we had a
"Girls Day" and Aunteee treated us to hour-long massages
that were truly needed. We then came home and had a
Birthday Party for my mom's caregiver and good friend
Kelly. She's been an awesome addition to my mother's
care and the two of them have forged a great friendship.

It was a memorable night full of love and laughter.
Between Aunteee cutting a step to The Average White
Band, a few sips of wine and beer, and an Extended
Version of Stevie Wonder's Happy Birthday song, it was
great to see mommy smiling and enjoying herself.

11. UNH REUNION *(2/14/10)*

This experience has reminded me of the great friends I
have acquired throughout my life. From the visits, calls,
flowers, and cards both my mom and I have received
from MY friends, it's an amazing feeling! Mom and I had a
visit today from two of my closest College friends. It was a
reunion for the ages because we haven't all been together
since one of their weddings several years ago. Time truly
does fly. They drove from New Hampshire and Boston to
simply hang out with us for a few hours and it truly
meant the world to both of us. I love those two ladies
more than they could ever know!

12. TATOOOOO (2/22/10)

I did it! On Friday I got tatted. This is my second tattoo and it's extremely important to me. I'm a firm believer that a tattoo is not something that should be taken lightly and if you're going to get one, it should have special significance to you. I mean after all, it IS permanent! One of my dear friends is a phenomenal artist and inspired the design. She put so much love and intricate detail into the original design that the tattoo artist said that it would have to be the size of an 8x11 piece of paper. I'm bold but not that bold, so he made some adjustments to bring it down to size but it was her interpretation of my request that made it turn out so beautifully.

My tattoo is a Lotus Flower for obvious reasons, with the Breast Cancer Pink Ribbon incorporated into it. It's abstract and truly a piece of art that I am proud to wear for the rest of my life in honor of my mother. I went home for a quick trip this weekend and unveiled it to my mom and she thinks it's beautiful. She even caught the tattoo bug but I kindly let her know that she may want not want to worry about it. After I described the pain, she quickly became de-bugged!

I debated back and forth on where I wanted it to be located and finally settled on my right side over my ribs for various reasons. I'm very happy with my decision. This just so happens to be the most painful place to get a tattoo according to my tattoo artist who let me know after he started! He was awesome and cracked a few jokes to help the time go by. It was uncomfortable and quite painful in a couple spots but overall it was bearable. I kept thinking to myself that the pain I was feeling was temporary and had no comparison to what my mother has been bearing. It made the moment a lot more somber and I got through it tear free! My boyfriend was there the entire time offering his hand for me to squeeze, which I did extremely hard! He was gracious and the moral support was more than appreciated.

13. AND SO IT BEGINS *(2/26/10)*

Mom has been holding up well since the radiation stopped about a month ago. It's been a blessing to see her improve and I've truly cherished the second chance I was given before the inevitable. I knew that the improvements would be short lived and kept that in the back of my head to enjoy our time. Sadly the decline has started. Mom has fallen three times in the last week and will be going back to the wheelchair. We booked a 5-day cruise for March 13th and I'm a little anxious about how she'll fare on it. She really wants to go so I respect her wishes, and we'll have fun together, but I'd be lying if I said I wasn't hesitant about the idea from its inception.

My dad is taking mom to Georgia to stay with my Aunteee and Uncle on Sunday. I have a very strong feeling that she will remain there. For that reason, I've been skittish about her going. I know it's best for her because both my aunt and uncle are retired and she'll have round the clock care. However, I know deep in my heart that this is the beginning of the last chapter and it hurts. As crazy as it sounds, I feel like if she stayed in Albany she'd stay with us longer. But that's selfish and I must let that go.

With this transition about to take place, my eyes have been opened to some things. Through this process, I've seen the absolute best in people and our true friends who have gone out of their way to visit, call, cook, and send a note or flowers. I also find myself irritated with people who love to hear themselves talk and demonstrate no follow up. I will not allow that negativity to overshadow the positive but be clear that I see you and know who you are. I need to vent here because its been building and I'll be damned if I let Laquita tear up another phone.

So consider this a Public Service Announcement. I could give a damn about how many times you tell me how much my mom has done for you or means to you if you can't take it upon yourself to pick up the phone to call her and tell her yourself. Don't tell her or me for that matter that you're coming to visit and then not only don't come but give no courtesy call. I could give a flying fuck about YOUR "grieving process" when it comes MY mother!! The last thing I want to hear is that you can't call or visit MY mother because it hurts YOU too much! You're bullshit, and will get thoroughly cussed out! For the rest of your life, you can deal with knowing that you were given the opportunity to do and say the right thing but chose not to! I'm so very glad I got that off my chest!

14. GEORGIA *(3/2/10)*

So mom is officially in Georgia now. My parents stopped in Baltimore yesterday in route and it was a numbing experience. As I stated in my last post, mom's decline has begun and it's rapid. Literally in a week's time she's back in the wheelchair. My house is not wheelchair accessible and that was never more evident than last night. Mom had to be lifted in my house because she couldn't get up my three front stairs. My boyfriend even had to stay overnight to help my father carry her out of my house this morning, as I'm no longer able to help lift her.

When she originally declined during radiation treatment she still had her leg strength so I could help her stand by myself. With this new turn of events she can't stand on her own at all as her legs buckle and I'm not physically capable of holding all of her weight. I give my father a ton of credit because he's the one who's been getting her around and it's not easy. Looking at her, it shows that her left side is the weaker of the two as even sitting straight up is difficult because she can't help but lean to the left. To put it frankly, it sucks to see my mother have to go through this TWICE. However, the first time mentally prepared me for this round.

The issue now is if she'll be able to even go on the cruise on the 13th. She's declined so rapidly, it seems like an impossible feat. Not only will she be on a ship in the middle of the ocean for 5 days, but she also has to be driven down to Miami from Georgia, which is a 13-hour drive because the doctor's won't clear her to fly. Couple this with the fact that it takes two men to get her in and out of the car currently and it will be just my aunt and me. My aunt is of the mindset that as long as mom's breathing, she's going on the cruise. I already know that we're going to bump heads on this. It's ultimately up to mom so I'm just laying low with my opinion to see how she fares over the next week.

Surprisingly, after today's whirlwind, I'm okay. My parents got to my house at 12am and I had to wake them up at 4:30am so they could get back on the road and they left at 5:45am. I kept my smile on for her and she had a few jokes once we got her settled in. Her spirit is good although I can look in her eyes and see that mentally, physically, and spiritually she's tired. I honestly don't blame her.

I'm past the point of selfishly wanting her to stay here as long as she can. I'm not the person who thinks that simply being alive or breathing with no quality of life is living. My mother is so much more than that. I really want her to be at peace. This illness has taken from my mother things that the average woman holds dear and she's taken it like a champ. She's lost her hair, both breasts, and to see her have to lose her mobility and function because of the cancer spreading to her brain is heartbreaking.

I'm going to miss her beyond my imagination but if it means she doesn't have to fight this bitch of a disease anymore, I'll let her go. Because at the end of the day, no matter what cancer has thrown at her, she never let it break her and for that, she's already won this battle. Her reward is way beyond this life and her legacy is vast. I'm tearing up as I'm typing this and although prepared for this part of the journey, I know that the toughest days are still to come. I would not wish this on my worst enemy.

If you're blessed to have your parents alive and well in your life, don't take it for granted! Don't let a single day go by without letting them know how much you love them!

15. CRUISIN' *(3/13/10)*

Well somehow through the grace of God we made it to Miami for the cruise later on today. I haven't slept yet since flying in at midnight. I'm completely overwhelmed by a tidal wave of different emotions. I've been attempting to mentally prepare myself to see my mother all week. I could tell from her speech or lack thereof over the phone how I thought she was faring. I haven't had a real conversation with my mom since she left Albany because of her condition and it's unnerving. I guess it's preparation for the inevitable but it still sucks nonetheless.

To see my mother today broke my heart and I actually had to step out of the room to get my bearings. She was sleeping when I arrived and incoherent from the pain meds. That smiling face that I'm so used to seeing couldn't respond to me. Mom can't hold herself up anymore or even turn herself over in bed. I strategically figured out how to turn her over on my own and as bad as she wanted to help me she couldn't. I'll hear her moan in discomfort and when I ask her what I can do she can barely get it out. I'd rather stay awake all night just so I can be alert to help her the best I can. Imagine that for a moment to step into my hurt right now. I haven't even seen the half yet. This is just her lying in bed. I'm blown.

My dad gave me a good pep talk this week even though he's going through his own emotions of coming home to an empty house. I'm going to make the most of this cruise and make it memorable. Every ounce of strength mom has left has been for this. She'll be able to spend quality time with My Aunteee, Cousin and I and get to visit my Grandmother in Jamaica for a day. It's what she wants and I'm going to do my absolute best to keep her smiling. This is not a rest and relaxation vacation for me more than an opportunity to show her all the love I can and I'm going to work hard doing it. If I hardly sleep then so be it. I can sleep when we get back.

The reality of what is coming has never been more apparent than what I'm seeing right now. There's no more promise of improvement. There's no more plateau. It's simply decline now...but I still feel her Spirit. This cruise is a rite of passage in more ways than one which is why I've been so apprehensive about it. But it's here and so are we, together, which is still a Blessing.

16. WE'RE BAAAACK *(3/21/10)*

So, the cruise came and went. So much has happened during and since that I'm trying to figure out where to begin. First and foremost, Royal Caribbean is an amazing cruise line. Our ship was phenomenal, the service was top notch, and it was definitely a time to remember with lots of memories made. Now with all that said, it was work! I went in with the right expectations for this trip and considered it a working vacation because we were able to do both. Each had their moment and when the moment came we worked really hard or let really loose!

I am so proud of mom! She held up so well and was the greatest trooper through everything. Aunteee gave my cousin and I a crash course on caregiving and we picked up quickly. Let's be clear. This caregiving is completely different from anything I thought I was doing before. Mom was lifted, held up, turned over, fed, wheeled, and beyond. My aunt is meticulous and she has been taking great care of my mother. With that great care comes a lot of work. Aunteee was and is the captain of the SS Caregiver when it comes to mom. We willingly took orders and proactively offered help. It was the perfect balance. If my cousin hadn't come on the cruise with us, I genuinely have no idea how we would have managed as mom has become completely dependent.

The climax of the trip was docking in Jamaica. The main reason we went on the cruise was so mom would be able to see my grandmother on my dad's side one last time. They are extremely close. Since she can't fly, a ship was the only way we were going to get there.

When we arrived in Jamaica, we were stressed because getting mom into the van to get to grandma's and then actually getting her up the front stairs of the house once we got there was going to be a struggle. But once again, the testament of how good God is came through. My uncle showed up in a bus he was able to borrow with a portable ramp that could be used for the house steps as well. All he had to do was roll mom on board and we were good to go.

Seeing my mom and grandma together instantly choked me up. I've seen my grandmother cry twice in my life. Once when my grandfather passed away and second when she saw my mother this last time. Grandma had the pastor from her church come by and we had prayer followed by lunch. We were able to spend a little over two hours with her before heading back to ship. It was definitely too short but those two hours meant everything to my mother.

It was bittersweet because sadly that was one of the last times I saw mom truly engaged with us. After Jamaica, mom was completely over the cruise and rightly so. She held up way longer than anyone could have expected her to. Since then, her decline has kicked back in. It seems now that she's had the opportunity to see those who meant the most to her, she's ready. She doesn't really talk more than a word here and there though she can still understand what you're saying to her and responds with a very low whisper or nod. Use of her legs went a couple weeks ago and now her arms are becoming weak as well. The new issue is her difficulty swallowing. This just started yesterday and is worrisome because she's struggling to take her essential medication. Come Monday, we'll have to find out options from her doctor down here in Georgia.

In spite of all that, mom cracked me a smile yesterday. It made my day and at the same time reminded me how much I'm going to miss it. I'm here in Georgia until Tuesday to help Aunteee out. My dad and Kelly are coming down in the morning from Albany to visit and it will be nice for all of us to be together again. I already know that leaving Tuesday is going to be the hardest departure of them all so far for me. I'll cross that bridge when I get there.

17. LETTING GO *(3/23/10)*

This is it. Mom was entered into Hospice Care at Aunteee's house today. It's been an exhausting 72 hours. I've been sleeping (at least attempting to) in the hospital with her the last two nights. I only left her side for 2 hours because my dad made me go to the house and take a nap on Monday. Otherwise, I just can't leave her.

My mother's difficulty swallowing forced us to take her to the Emergency Room on Sunday shortly after my dad and Kelly arrived. After a slew of blood work, x-rays, and CT Scans, we found out that my mom's cancer has also spread to both lungs and that it was time to plan for Hospice. While heartbroken, I wasn't surprised. I already knew in my heart that the cruise was one of the last things mom wanted to do. I also knew that once we returned she would begin to let go...but Damn. We JUST got back on Thursday and it's only Tuesday! I thought I would have more time! It wasn't supposed to happen this fast! I've been an emotional wreck these last three days. I don't want to talk to anyone unless they're already down here with me. I'm simply trying to process this shit and honor my mother's wishes.

Mom appointed me her Health Care Proxy. It's a huge responsibility and a lot of pressure but I know she trusts me. She did a living will and her desires are clear...No Pain and DNR, in other words, Do Not Resuscitate. I want her to stay here but I can't in good conscience go against her wishes or prolong the inevitable, so I have to let her go and it hurts like hell.

In Georgia hospice, the main and only goal is to provide comfort from pain. There are no feeding tubes; no hydration IV's...nothing but pain meds. I'm watching my mother cross over and this is the hardest thing I've ever had to do in my life. She mostly sleeps, unless she's having breakthrough pain where she can get very active with her arms to let us know she's hurting, but mom being mom has given us some inspiration along the way.

The first night in the ER, the doctors warned me that because my mother's blood pressure was so low, if they give her pain meds and she stopped breathing I would need to make a decision about resuscitating her. What the fuck?!?! Everyone had just gone home for the night and here I am, simply wanting to comfort my mother who was writhing in pain because she couldn't swallow her pain pills and now if I did she could die?! I freaked the hell out!

Through my tears, I asked my mom for help because I didn't know what to do. I told her I was doing my best, and that I loved her. In her pain, and altered mental state, her face became calm, she squeezed my hand, and she looked me in my eyes. She couldn't speak but I knew what she was saying. I called everyone back so that when they administered her pain medication, if it took her under, at least they could be there. She fought through that.

Today my grandmother from Jamaica called and my aunt put her on speakerphone. My mother, who hasn't spoken since Saturday, called out "Mom Mom" when she heard her voice...and I missed it! I was in the dining room being forced to eat lunch when it happened, but it's those little things that keep giving us hope through this painful process.

I asked the hospice nurse how long she believed my mother had today. She told me 2-3 days. Can you believe that shit? This time last week we were on the cruise! I will say this. The power of the mind is phenomenal. My mother fought her cancer tooth and nail to get on that ship so she could see my grandmother in Jamaica. She maintained herself while on the cruise and once it was official that the cruise was over, she let it all go. She was the epitome of determination and her strength amazes me.

I'm sitting at her side now as I type this and hearing her breath is the sweetest sound. I really can't believe that this is it. I've talked, blogged, prayed, thought it over and still can't wrap my mind around the fact that this time next week, I'm going to want to call my mom and won't be able to because I'll be planning her Home Going Celebration. She's only 55 and up to last week this time was full of life and smiles in spite of her condition. I have NO idea where to go from here...

18. A NEW CHAPTER *(4/13/10)*

Brenda Carol Walters

Sunrise 8/31/54-Sunset 3/24/10

On March 24th 2010, at approximately 3:30am, my Best Friend, Hero, and Mother, earned her wings and passed over. I knew the time was coming. I honestly didn't know it was going to happen so quickly. Mommy passed away two hours after I wrote the last chapter. It's surreal to read it now because at the time when I wrote it I had no idea she was so close to leaving me (in the physical sense). I remember wanting to stay with her for as long as I could that night because the two previous nights at the hospital had been so stressful. That coupled with the news we had received from the Hospice nurse earlier that day, I was completely unsettled. Writing that night was a way for me to stay awake as long as I could.

I was awakened at 3:00am by activity in mommy's room that was next to mine. Her breathing was extremely labored. My dad, aunt, and mom's friend were tending to her, as it was time for her to get her pain medication. I'll never forget that sound. I had spent so much time listening for her breath because of the hospital scare and this was different from anything I had ever heard. I called the on call hospice nurse and she calmly let me know that mommy was preparing to cross over. Stunned, we gave her her pain medication and shortly after, her breathing slowed significantly. Within twenty minutes, I saw my dad take off her oxygen mask and that was it. She went home peacefully. All the preparation in the world did not prepare me for that moment...or the days following.

Once mommy passed, my dad and I went into business mode making preparations for her Home Going and Memorial Services. All went smoothly and mom's life and legacy were celebrated although none of it was easy. The funeral was held down in Warner Robins Georgia, as it was my mother's request to be laid to rest down there. Although a blur, I specifically remember my tears, the music, the eulogy getting the church on their feet, and the burial. I remember having to be pulled away from her casket at the cemetery because I simply wasn't going to leave her out there. After the interment, I stood there with my hand touching the casket and I was frozen. I believe it was my dad who pulled me away and once back in the limo I remember breaking down and feeling the helpless energy of those in the car who wanted to help me so badly but knew that I was inconsolable at that moment.

I also remember how mom looked in the casket. Pictures were taken of her but I haven't seen them nor am I sure if I ever want to. The image is seared in my brain and I'll never forget it. It was of the utmost importance to me that she looked like herself. I had been to viewings in the past where the makeup was too much or didn't match and

that simply wasn't going to happen with my mother. I'll
never forget having to decide along with Aunteee which
one of mom's dresses we were going to choose. I
remember having to buy her a new wig, a scarf for her
dress, earrings, a bracelet and nail polish. I remember
going through her makeup for the last time choosing
what to give the mortician and reminiscing of the days
when I would play dress up with her clothes, and shoes as
a child. I even gave the mortician a picture of mom before
she was put on the steroids because a side effect was that
it added weight to her face. Mommy was always fierce
and her last viewing would be no different. She looked so
peaceful and as I wished she looked like Brenda. It was
the craziest feeling to be mortified that I'm looking at my
mother in a casket yet at the same time relieved that the
mortician ensured that she looked like her beautiful self.

The church in Albany for the Memorial Service was
standing room only. There weren't as many tears at the
memorial service on my part. I believe at that point I was
quasi cried out and numb, but the service had a more
celebratory feeling to it since mommy had already been
laid to rest. I remember music again and very kind words.
I remember being overwhelmed by the number of people
who came to show their respect and remind my dad and I
how much mom impacted them for the better. Although
the energy in the sanctuary was sad and somber it was
also beautiful because it was filled with love.

Now that the whirlwind is over, it's time to settle into some sense of normalcy, but there's one huge piece of the puzzle missing and we miss her so much. I'm settled with the fact that mom was ready and we weren't. I'm settled with the fact that she did everything she wanted to do and went home on her terms. I'm settled with the fact that she's at peace and no longer has to deal with the pain that came from breast cancer and this world. I'm settled with the fact that I took full advantage of the time I was blessed to have with her and there was no question in her mind of my love and adoration for her. I'm settled with the fact that I have the best Guardian Angel anyone could ask for. I'm settled with the fact that her life and legacy live through me and I will continue to make her proud. I'm settled!!! None of that changes the fact that I MISS HER! I want nothing more than to pick up the phone and hear her voice and to walk in her room and see her Big, Bright Smile followed with a hug that only she could give. I'm more blown by the fact that if I'm blessed to have a long life, I'll have had more years here without her than with her.

All that being said, I'm on One Day at a Time status. Some days are better than others and as I write this new chapter that's all I know to do. I debated over continuing to write now that mommy's gone, but as the days progress, this part of the journey is just as significant. Getting the emotions out can't hurt more than help. I'm Brenda's Daughter so I have no choice but to overcome in the long run. However, the process is going to be just that.

19. BUT GRACE *(4/18/10)*

This week was interesting. On my "one day at a time" status, I made it through the week without crying. I'd have random waves of sadness but no tears. I spoke to my dad and my aunteee and they both expressed having pretty tough weeks dealing with mom's passing. As I thought about it, I realized that being here in Baltimore, I'm detached from certain aspects of mommy being gone. My dad now has an empty house to go to everyday and since my mom passed and was laid to rest in Georgia, aunteee has a direct connection as well that I don't have here.

Then Saturday came, and that feeling I've come to know so well overwhelmed me. I woke up heavy. I went to brunch with my one of my friend's hoping to take my mind off of things and it helped a little. But by the time I got home, I watched a couple videos of mom, welled up a little and went to sleep. If I had my way, I'd sleep most of the time because it seems that it's only then that I don't have to think about the obvious. I actually slept for the rest of the afternoon. Only for the sake of my boyfriend coming over did I even force myself to get out of bed.

I find myself pretty indifferent these days. Not much of anything overly excites me or irritates me. Both sides of the coin seem pointless right now. If something gets on my nerves, it's not worth my time to let it fester like I used to (which might actually be a positive). On the other hand, the things that I used to get excited about are just cool. Things I would do a happy dance for before are now just, blah. I'm simply content to make it through the day without a breakdown.

I forced myself to get up and go to church today and I will say that it helped but the first part of the service was rocky and I almost walked out. Within five minutes of sitting down in the sanctuary, the drama ministry was doing a presentation and in the play the character was diagnosed with cancer (if you could have seen the look on my face). Next was the altar call and the pastor had a young man testify about how his mom passed away in 2008 (cue in breakdown). I'm sitting in the pew sobbing/borderline wailing because the entire purpose of me forcing myself to go to church was to be encouraged and take my mind OFF of the hurt. Lord I know I looked crazy. Thank God for the lady next to me. She just rubbed my back and comforted me. I wanted to leave so badly but I couldn't get out of my seat...and I'm so glad that I didn't.

The sermon was perfect for me. I was reminded about all the things that God has brought me through and how He's never left me. I was reminded that He's still with me during this time of bereavement, and that even when I was expected to stumble and fall, if I did, I didn't stay down. This walk is no different. I was able to release a praise that was deep down in my spirit today because of that, and it felt great! That doesn't make moving forward any easier but it gives me encouragement. I came home afterwards, uplifted, not completely out of my funk but higher than when I left my house that morning.

The pastor talked a lot about needing your space when life knocks you down. My funk is my need of space. I appreciate the love, prayers, and support. I genuinely know that they are working. But this is a journey that is only mine. While there are people who can empathize, and may have lost a parent, not one person can know what my mom meant to me and how deeply this loss affects me nor can I know what their parent or loved one meant to them. I'm not supposed to. With that, I'll choose my words carefully from now on when I say, "I know what you're going through". The art of this new chapter for me is balancing the need to have my space with knowing when to lean on those close to me for help and support. All I can say is, I'm learning. I have another day under my belt and I'll take it.

20. THE NOT SO OBVIOUS *(4/24/10)*

I was ripped from my sleep at 5:57 this morning because of a dream about my dad. I'm never up this early...especially on a Saturday, but it messed with me that much. I honestly can't remember the last time I dreamt about my dad so vividly. I called him to check in on him and he said he was okay but I just couldn't go back to sleep so I'm here. The other part that's making my mind work overtime is that my mom had the ability to dream about people. I remember in college, she would call me up and simply say, "What are you doing"...not as a question but as a statement and it always happened when I was doing something I shouldn't have been doing or losing focus. Those calls use to freak me out! Since mommy passed, my dreams have been getting more vivid and I wonder if that's something else that she passed on to me. We'll see...

My dream was all over the place but it took me from a party to a sanctuary full of old church members from when I was a little girl in Rochester NY, some of my cousins from Georgia and other random people. An argument broke out between two ladies that I don't know and then my dad came storming down the church aisle fussing about something and I heard him mention my mom. I went after him outside and we both started to cry remembering her. It was in the dream that I realized, everyone was so worried about me and how I would handle mom's passing, that no one really considered him.

We walked and talked in my dream until we both calmed down a little, and at that point I woke up.

My parents were married for 33 years. That's a long time to love, live with, and know somebody. That's longer than I've been alive! Their relationship had its ups and downs over the years but my dad was the only one who was there everyday during mommy's nine-year off and on battle with breast cancer. As much as I wanted to be there, I couldn't be there the way he was because I live in Baltimore. He was always the liaison between my mom and her close friends and family when she would at times understandably shut them out. He's the reason my mom and aunteee mended their strained relationship. He knew and understood her in a way that even I didn't back when she was first diagnosed. He was holding her hand when she passed away. Even with all that known, it never dawned on me how hard mommy's passing would hit him. I don't even think he realized it because him and mom always concerned themselves with me first. I remember right after she passed, I heard him whisper to her that he was always going to take care of me and that I would be okay.

At mom's services, my dad made a statement that I never heard him say before. He said that people need not to focus on the last nine years where he was mom's primary caregiver but on the previous 25 years that she helped him become the man he is today. He mentioned that she was the epiphany in his life that turned him around and put him on the right path. I never knew that. That's when I realized how much she really meant to him and how much he truly loved her. No matter what was going on, they could be working each other's last nerve, but he ALWAYS showed up. He walked with her everyday and that says a lot, especially in this day and age when people bail on marriage so quickly. To go from that to her being gone would be clearly devastating. This coupled with the fact that he has the empty house to now go to everyday. I mentioned in the last chapter that as much as I have my ups and downs, I'm still somewhat detached because I'm not in Albany NY where they lived. Because of that, in my delusional mind, I can trick myself into thinking that I simply haven't spoken to her in a couple of days.

All that brought me to this thought...while my dad and I are grieving for the loss of the same person, we're grieving differently and for different reasons. Leaning on each other will be the only way that we both stay standing. My heart hurts for him because he lost his best friend too. My parent's pastor pulled me aside while we were in Georgia right before mom's home going service. He told me a story about when he, my dad, and few of the fellas were out golfing. One of the guy's wives kept calling him and borderline harassing him while they were on the golf course. This prompted a discussion about marriage, relationships etc and he told me that my dad said he had the best in my mom. What was so moving about this statement was that this was amongst men so my dad could've been brutally honest and whatever was said would've stayed there. Yet he chose to say that. Simply put, that's love.

Well as part of my process, I booked an impromptu trip to Jamaica to visit with my grandmother. She's another one who's been taking mom's passing pretty hard. She tells me every time I talk to her that my mom wasn't just a daughter in law, she was a daughter. I start a new career on May 3rd, which I'm extremely excited about. However, having to stay in this house for another week would cause me to lose my mind. Too much time on my hands to sit around and think is not a good thing so as of tomorrow I will be in Jamaica! I'm going alone which I've never done before, but I think it'll be good for grandma and me.

21. THE MASK *(5/4/10)*

"We wear the mask that grins and lies. It hides our cheeks
and shades our eyes. This debt we pay to human guile;
with torn and bleeding hearts we smile..."
~Paul Laurence Dunbar~

One Day At A Time. This poem depicts how I feel on a day-to-day basis. I've always loved this poem since I first read it in college. It rings no truer than right now in my life. I wake up everyday...and everyday since March 24th is a new day without her. Wednesdays are the toughest because that's the day she passed. Sundays I release all the tears I held in for the most part that week at church. Everyday in between I'm seemingly okay. I'm smiling, laughing, joking around even...simply covering my reality because if I honestly walked around the way I truly felt inside, no one would want to be around me. I don't think I'd want to even be around myself. So I wear the mask. The issue about the mask is that it unexpectedly falls off from time to time and without warning, the sadness that I carry with me but bury daily emerges like the snap of a finger leaving those in my presence feeling awkward because I may have been smiling moments earlier. These moments usually happen when I'm alone but every once in a while I'm reminded that as much as I try to control my emotions, they're still going to get the best of me at times. And there's currently nothing I can do about it.

Jamaica was exactly what I needed. I came back fully recharged. I did nothing but relax, eat, drink, go to the beach, read, and sleep. Grandma was shocked to see me hanging around the house so much and not "bleaching" so she calls it when we hang out late, but I know it meant a lot to her as it did me. We sat on the veranda a lot. Sometimes we talked a mile a minute and sometimes we just sat there enjoying the sea breeze and each other's company. She repeated everyday that mommy wasn't just a daughter in law but a daughter. I swear I could feel her with us on the veranda in the breeze at times but then again I wonder if my mind was playing tricks on me.

Mommy had such a huge spirit, I often imagined before she passed that even after she was gone in the physical I'd still be able to talk to her. I imagined that she would come to me in my dreams or that I could hear her still voice in my ear. Unfortunately, those events haven't happened, and I really miss her. I talk out loud when I'm alone just to tell her that I miss her. I'll even spray her perfume on my pillows at night sometimes to remind me of her and to hopefully summon her into my dreams. It sounds crazy I'm sure but it's those little things that still keep her close to me even though she's not here. I know now that my mother was fully prepared to leave here and put parameters in place that my dad and I didn't even know about financially to ensure that we would be okay. However we would give it ALL back just to have her here with us. Her presence was unmatched!

I started my new job yesterday and really believe that it's a great fit for me. As excited as I was after my first day, I was humbled because I wasn't able to call the first person I normally would have. You simply don't understand how much my mother supported me. She was always so excited for me when a new opportunity arose, if not excited more than me. I can hear her voice now saying, "I know that's right shawty!". We would've joked and sang silly songs on the phone and she would have told me how proud she was of me. How everything I went through getting laid off last year prepared me for this great opportunity. How I was going to be the Number 1 Sales Rep. When I was growing up, whenever I had a solo, performance, track meet etc and she was able to make it, she always made her presence known. "That's my baby!", I can hear her say or "Sannnng Riss!". It always put a smile on my face. It hurts to know that I won't hear that voice again.

So today the mask came off unexpectedly as I pulled out mommy's beloved All God's Children figurines. They were her pride and joy. My house isn't big enough to hold the entire collection she had so I kept some signature pieces that I knew were really special to her and gave the majority to my Aunteee who has the room to display them as well as some other family and friends that I knew would appreciate them. Before I knew it, the tears came and I couldn't fight it. So as I go to sleep tonight, I'll pick out a new mask to wear tomorrow because the one I wore today broke in the fall. We'll see how long this one lasts.

22. SHE KNEW OF A BETTER PLACE *(5/9/10)*

What a weekend! I figured that Mother's Day weekend would be a little difficult but it was a lot more difficult than I imagined. It's par for the course I guess, and a part of my journey. But I definitely wasn't prepared. Friday night presented my seemingly cyclical melt down. It seems to happen once every couple of months. The bitterness, anger, and rage that I keep in check day to day overwhelm me. It came out of nowhere but it was building. I was just really hurting and missing mom.

It started when I received a picture of the marker on her gravesite via text message on Friday morning. It takes over a month for the marker to be put in place. It finally arrived at some point last week unbeknownst to me and I wasn't forewarned of the image that came to my phone. It happened while at work and my heart sank but I was in business mode so I couldn't and didn't show emotion at the time. I actually didn't realize how much it affected me until Friday night and by then it was too late.

I watched the DVD of pictures of mommy that was played at her memorial services on repeat that night and the waterfall of tears came. It was just all too much. I called my dad and we had a talk that I will never forget. He did for me what my mom had done for me all these years. All throughout my life, whenever I had a breakdown, be it regarding my career, relationships and everything in between, mommy was the FIRST person I called. She would always "bring me back". I'd be a blubbering mess when I called her and she would be the one to calm me down, stop the tears, and pray for me over the phone until I fell asleep.

My dad stepped in that night and filled her role to a tee. We talked for a while. He said some really profound things and reminded me that my journey and struggle was not mine alone. There's a bond that we share through this transition that's only for us to understand. He told me that one of the things he holds onto is that my mother KNEW there was a better place for her. She NEVER questioned that. It explains a lot about her final days and how she carried herself. She had a peace that I will always remember. He said that if she knew there was a better place for her, then we needed to believe that same thing and exude the same faith she did. He then prayed with me over the phone just like mommy would have and before I knew it I was sleeping. A blubbering mess when I called him, my dad brought me back.

Saturday was hot and cold. I was busy with errands and events to attend so I didn't have time to completely focus on the hurt. Yet I still had my moments. It was my dad's birthday and he sent ME a gift card to help take my mind off things. I can't help but love that man! It's definitely the little things that help along the way. Today was okay. I chose to isolate myself, which I believe was the best remedy for me. I didn't want to go to brunch surrounded by people celebrating with their mothers knowing that I couldn't. I didn't want to go to church because I just didn't want to break down again and I knew it was inevitable on a day like today. My boyfriend surprised me with a sweet gift to lift my spirits and then we went to the mall for a little retail therapy. Exhausted from this emotionally draining weekend I came back to the house and slept for three hours. I woke up at 8:30pm happy that the day was almost over and that I made it.

I remember my mother fondly today. I remember her faith, her praise, her spirit, her strength, her grace, her wisdom, her kind heart, her voice, her discernment, and her willingness to help anyone who needed it. I miss her presence like nothing I've ever known but I know that she only left here because she knew that I would be in good hands. Her will wouldn't have allowed her to leave if she didn't believe that. So I have another day under my belt and I'm hurt but not broken. Mommy wouldn't let anything break her and that strength resides in me.

23. BEEN GONE FOR A MINUTE *(6/29/10)*

It's been a while but I really needed to take a break and shift my energy to a more positive place. Writing has been my sounding board throughout this difficult transition and as a result it's very heavy. I pride myself on trying to stay positive and looking back over my previous blog entries is very bittersweet as I go right back to the place I was physically, mentally and emotionally per chapter. For obvious reasons they are the darkest moments of my life and while it's good to know where I've come from, I believe the purpose of life is to never dwell in the dark but to learn and in your best attempt, eventually move forward back to the light.

A lot has happened since my last chapter, which was a tough one, and it's all happened without my mom by my side physically, but I know she's with me. At least in my heart of hearts I believe it and it keeps me going. She still hasn't presented herself to me in my dreams and that hurts because I just knew she would dwell there to keep me company. Yet and still, I keep hope alive for that. I have a few coping mechanisms that help and I'd like to share them as they're all part of the journey.

First, I never leave the house without wearing something that belonged to my mother, which is always a piece or two of her jewelry. I feel protected by her this way. Case in point, on Saturday evening I was out with my girlfriends and being scatterbrained which is something that tends to happen more frequently as of late, I left my phone sitting at the bar, went to another floor in the venue and not until about 30 minutes later realized it was missing. Frantic, I ran back to the bar and sure enough the bartender had it and said that "someone" turned it in. Ironic maybe but it makes me wonder. Second, retail therapy has been a big help. I'm much wiser with money than I was when I was younger and that's definitely thanks to her. Mommy always taught me to treat myself first. Let's just say that I've been doing a lot of treating to make myself feel better. It's never long lived but it helps when I need it. Third, I still occasionally spray her perfume on my pillows before I go to sleep. Fourth, is my newfound fascination with the moon at night.

On a clear night I can find myself fixated and completely lost in thought staring at the moon and wondering what's past it. I speculate about what's on the other side and if I'll accomplish all that I want and need to before I'm allowed to see it and see her again. I realize how small I really am in the grand scheme of things and how in passing my mother transformed into something so much bigger than my little mind can imagine. Is she with me 24/7 or is she caught up getting her praise on in heaven? Or better yet, is she doing both simultaneously?

I've lost loved ones before but never before have I been so consumed with what's going on on the other side than now since she's not here. There are so many questions I

want to ask her in my dreams like: What's heaven like?
Did I do a good job in your final days? Can you see my
future? How will I be the manifestation of your legacy?
How big is the universe? Did you get to see the world
before you crossed over? Do you get to see the world
now? What's your favorite place? Are you looking down
on me from Heaven or are you down here with me and
can go back and forth? Were you the one who ensured
that when I didn't fully close my front door leaving it
partially open in the city of Baltimore that no one came
inside my house and robbed me blind? Those questions
are just the tip of the iceberg.

 I'm remembering why I stopped writing for a bit as I well
up with tears writing this. However, if I didn't let them
out now, they'd come out later so there's no point in
holding them in. All in all, I'm hanging in there. I'm
laughing more now and trying to figure this "new me" out.
My new career is keeping me really busy which is
wonderful for my sanity. So between that, prayer, retail
therapy, writing, my new fascination with the moon and
my little rituals, I'm okay. At this point that's all I can be
and I'm good with that.

24. PRUNING *(7/6/10)*

This journey has been full of twists, turns and unknowns. Everyday is a new day to fight through and for the most part I win or draw. But sometimes I lose. Today I lost. What many people don't understand is this process is just that...a process. My frustration is finding that most people have moved on with their lives since my mother passed while my Father, Aunteee, Kelly and I are still working through every single day. While many people can look at us and say, "it's been three months", our response is "it's ONLY been three months". My father told me today that I couldn't judge people for not being as attached to mom's passing as we are. For him to say that said a lot because I try my best to be a non-judgmental individual but I was doing just that. Not necessarily because they have obviously moved on but for treating me as if I should have too and unfortunately I've grown to resent those individuals.

Everyday I still grieve. I may not show it but I do. From wanting to call her because something great happened, or wanting to talk to her because I need guidance. I'm learning to look within, as I know that her counsel resides there. However, what I've learned the hard way is that I need to focus on getting through this grieving process. If you don't help me, you hinder me. Hindering me keeps me in this "process" longer. I've tried to let people in. I've tried to explain repeatedly what I do and don't need. Unfortunately, if one genuinely doesn't grasp the concept then I have to let them go. I have to let them go because my well being in the long term is more important right now than having my hurt compounded with additional confusion and frustration. In that horrible place I stay stagnant and that is something I simply cannot do.

I've been told that I've changed. How could I not have? How could I possibly stay the same person without my best friend here to protect and guide me? That inherently happy-go-lucky woman I used to be has evaded me for some time now and it hurts. However, this change has made me more aware of my surroundings. It's allowed me to see what's healthy and what isn't. Things I didn't pay attention to before are glaring at me now and I can't ignore them.

I now understand that my expectations may have increased too rapidly for some of those close to me. While I'm changing, I expect those close to me to change as well or at the very least accept my change. Some of them didn't and I could no longer ignore it. As a result my tree is a little lighter today. I'm by no means happy about my loss but if I'm not in a healthy place, I have to move forward without. They say that in order to grow sometimes you need to cut a few branches. I'm not in the position anymore to teach people how to interact with me. I haven't had that patience since January 5th and I genuinely don't think I'll ever have it again.

I honestly feel better going through this transition alone. I fight the hurt of the loss of my mother everyday. I can't keep fighting outside factors as well. I miss Brenda now more than ever and it hurts that the person I thought was up to the task to walk with me wasn't. So I'll walk alone.

25. A NECESSARY STEP (7/27/10)

I've been working through my pruning process and staying busy with work, which keeps me levelheaded. The pruning process has not been an easy one as it currently compounds the hurt that I'm already feeling but in the end I know it's for the best. I had a great visit from mommy's friend Kelly about a week ago and we had a great time hanging out while laughing and crying over mommy's antics. Brenda was feisty and had no problem getting her point across when necessary. If her head ever cocked to the side, it was in your best interest to get out of the way!

As a little girl I remember when my mother worked part time at the Division For Youth in Rochester NY. DFY as it was referred to, was a home for at-risk youth. In typical Brenda fashion, her time there left a positive impression on the youth she worked with. My mother was tough. She didn't play around and earned the respect of the young people she came in contact with. She always had this unique way of balancing compassion with a no nonsense attitude. I'll never forget seeing pictures of the young men in different "jail pose" stances and then turning the picture over and seeing written ever so affectionately "Love you Mom". That was Brenda all day and one of hundreds of crazy stories about her!

My dad sent Kelly down because he's worried about me and I'm so glad he did. He told me during one of my breakdowns that mommy rarely made mistakes. We both know now that she knew way before we or the doctors knew that her time was coming to a close and she placed people in our lives that she knew would be there to help soften the blow of losing her. Kelly was one of those people as well as my Aunteee.

Through all of these changes, I've realized that seeking professional counseling for my grieving process was necessary and I went to my first session today. Let's just say I won't be going back to that particular counselor. Bless his heart, he tried but there was no "click" or chemistry. I was able to get a good cry out but as far as what I'm looking for in the realm of a structured process to help me get through this, he was clueless. I mean, can I get a book to read, an exercise, or something?! He told me what I already knew which is not why I want to give up my co-pay. I'll try again next month with someone new.

I'm beginning this week knowing that before it's over I'll be taking another necessary step and saying I'm not thrilled is putting it nicely. I have my family reunion in Warner Robins Georgia this weekend, which is bittersweet for multiple reasons. It will be great to see my family, specifically Aunteee and Unc; however, I'll also be seeing my mother's gravesite for the first time since the funeral. I'm all over the place emotionally because of that.

I definitely know that mommy is gone but there's confirmation at her gravesite that will make it much more real for me. I don't know if I'm ready but there's no way I can go down there and not visit her. I'm attempting to prepare myself mentally for that moment however, in my heart of hearts I know that there's nothing I can really do. I will simply have to figure it out once I'm in it as I've been doing thus far. This will by far be the most difficult step to take and unfortunately, I'll be traveling to Georgia solo.

It just seems like every time I get through a new milestone without her, there's another one popping up. I got through Mother's Day. I got through my birthday. I'm working through my current emotions and anger at the four-month point as I realize that she's really not coming back. I'll have her gravesite by week's end and as soon I work through that, I'll have her Birthday at the end of August and then the holidays are right around the corner. Ugh!! I feel like I'm always a step behind and that's frustrating because I'm traditionally a step ahead. But nevertheless, I must push forward...so I will.

26. MY EPIPHANY *(8/5/10)*

The trip to Georgia was bittersweet as expected but once again a necessary step on my path. It was great to see my family. It's amazing to walk in a room full of people that you don't know but feeling a sense of security because it's family. That was a sweet part. I stayed with my Aunteee and Unc during the visit and slept in the room mommy passed away in. I remember when she first passed away and sleeping in that room, I'd keep the light on. Not sure why but I did. This time around I slept with the lights off and for the first time I had a dream with her talking to me (or at least trying).

In my dream, someone handed me a phone and I could hear her on the other line. I was so excited!! I remember telling her how happy I was to hear her voice and how I never thought I'd hear it again! But I realized that she couldn't hear me. I could hear her asking if anyone was there but she couldn't hear my response. She then said that she would just go ahead and leave a message and as soon as she started the phone started breaking up! Ugh! I woke up frustrated but then joyful that I heard her and at least I knew she was trying to talk to me. That was another sweet part of the trip.

The bitter part was visiting mommy's gravesite for the first time since the funeral. Since I flew down to Georgia alone, I decided I'd go alone. My dad came down to

Georgia as well and offered to go with me but I declined. For me, there was a symbolism in my solo trip and I will never forget that even though it was a solo trip it didn't have to be. While going through my pruning process, my relationship with my boyfriend took an unexpected turn. I learned rather quickly that we didn't have the same expectations after my mother passed away and I began to resent him for it as we had been together for so long. I resented that it was seemingly so easy for him to move on. I resented that he had never even been to a funeral before my mother's so as a result he was ill equipped to know how to handle my grief. He hadn't experienced that type of loss let alone any significant loss firsthand when it pertained to death.

As a result, it seemed like he always wanted our relationship to go back to January 4th and wouldn't accept that that period of time was over and that woman is gone. I expected him to grow with me as I figured out this new me but it was as if he was frozen in time. So we broke up and are now in that weird reconciliation place. I requested that he come down with me because I genuinely didn't want to go to Georgia and face mommy's gravesite by myself but since I had, I did. That's the interesting part of the pruning process I guess. I know now that when pruning, you need to cut the entire branch but because this particular branch once bloomed it's much harder to nip it in the bud (pun intended). It's much easier said than done.

As expected, the first time I went to her gravesite, I broke down. Through my tears, I couldn't stop staring at it. I just stood there and cried. When I finally calmed down, I started looking around the cemetery and looking at the other sites. Some had little benches and additional decorations and as crazy as it sounds I felt this sense of competition thinking to myself there's No Way MY mommy's going to be out here and not be represented to the fullest! She's going to get a bench too and whatever else I can find! People walking by will know that my mother was loved and adored in life and passing! I have no clue why my mind went there but it did and I got so consumed with it I stopped crying all together. Perhaps it was a defense mechanism but regardless, I'm on a mission!

Something about being in the room my mom passed away in gave me peace and insight that I hadn't had throughout this journey. I can still feel her energy in there. I began to have a deeper understanding of the struggles that my mom faced on a daily basis with her battle with cancer and depression. She stood up to them all...everyday. However, I can only imagine the toll that takes on one's spirit as time continues and mommy battled for nine years! I can recall looking at her earlier in the year when she was still here and seeing how tired she was. I can also recall many times over the years her simple desire for peace.

I now understand that she wouldn't have gotten that peace here on earth. I now understand that she could've thrown the towel in years ago but she stayed here for nine more years because she loved me! Three bouts with breast cancer is no easy feat. She went through three separate experiences of different chemotherapies and radiation. She grew back and lost her hair three times. She had her breasts removed as a preventative measure to simply be told 7 months later that the cancer had come back...and she still fought. I understand it all now. It doesn't make me miss her any less but I truly, truly understand why she couldn't stay here anymore and I know in my heart of hearts that she stayed here as long as she did for me. I can continue to move forward in life knowing that my mother loved me hard, in spite of all the times she may not have felt it in her own life, and to have experienced that love in this life is more than enough for me. That's my epiphany.

27. HAPPY BIRTHDAY BRENDA *(8/31/10)*

Yet another milestone without her. It's a little after 12am on August 31st and it's officially what would have been mommy's 56th birthday. Since my last entry I can say that emotionally, I've been pretty even keel. I haven't had any emotional breakdowns or cry fests and it honestly feels weird. I'm definitely not "over it" but there's a sense of numbness that understands crying simply will not bring her back to me in the way that I want her here. What it *will* do is leave me with a headache, swollen eyes, runny nose, and emotionally drained. I simply don't have it in me to keep crying over a lost cause. It doesn't mean that I don't have waves of sadness here and there but it doesn't get much deeper than that right now. I've been anticipating the arrival of her birthday, not sure if this current state of emotion is simply a front for the tsunami that will inevitably hit me today, but 15 minutes in and so far so good.

I honestly feel like I get it now. Since my last post, I've carried that sentiment with me of knowing that mommy only stayed here for as long as she did because of her love for me and it keeps me in a safe place. I still miss her tremendously. I still wish I could talk to her knowing that she would help me iron out all of my relationship issues. I still would love to see her bright smile. I still yearn for her big hugs. I still long for her antics that used to drive me up the wall. But I keep every moment in my heart. She dwells there and I can feel her. My stance at this juncture is to live life fully. Mommy never got to see the world in her physical being so nestled in my heart; she'll see it through me. With that said, I'll be leaving for Paris on Friday! My first trip overseas besides Jamaica and I'm going solo...or as I affectionately put it: Me, Myself and I...and Brenda. I'll be in Paris for three days and then head to Rome and I cannot wait! I'm anxious and elated at the same time! This is a first for me but definitely not a last and I know that this trip will be life changing in a positive way.

My original thought was to simply get through mommy's birthday as fast as I could with no major fanfare. My new therapist however, suggested I write her a letter so that's what the remainder of this chapter will be.

Dear Mommy,

It's been a little over 5 months since you departed and I can honestly say that this has been the hardest year of my life. Although I can feel your presence sometimes, at other times you seem so far away. It's at those moments that I try to lean on the lessons you taught me. How you taught me to be independent. How you taught me to love myself even when I feel so far from the only one besides God who loved me the hardest. I know I've had moments that made you proud on this journey and I know I've had moments where you were disappointed because you taught me better. But please know that I'm only trying to find my way without you and sometimes I feel so lost. My

love and adoration for you hasn't changed. You're STILL
my BEST FRIEND. You're STILL the ONLY person who
truly gets me...in all of my glory and all of my
shortcomings. It hurts the most to think that I may never
have that connection again with another human being. I
hate having to explain myself to people. You always
understood. I miss how we could sit in a room or on the
phone and not say anything but say so much at the same
time. I can honestly say that I understand you now. There
were times when honestly I didn't and I want nothing
more than to hug you and tell you that I understand
everything. I know why you were tired. I know why you
simply wanted peace. I know why you couldn't stay here
and I appreciate you so much for staying here as long as
you did. I'll never truly know the love you had for me
until the day I'm blessed to have my own children and it
breaks my heart that I won't be able to look into your eyes
and share that confirmation. It's not fair that I can't have
you here but it wasn't fair for you to suffer for as long as
you did either. You are my heart and soul. You come
through my pores. People tell me all the time how I look
and sound like you and it makes me smile. I didn't get to
show you all the things I wanted to, nor did I get to spoil
you and shower you with all the things you deserved but
together, we'll do it. I choose to live for both of us. I'm
going to live fully and I'm going to love hard. I will do
everything you wanted to do but couldn't knowing that
you're with me. I wish I could call you and sing you the
goofy Happy Birthday song we always sang to each other
but I must settle for this letter. However, I won't settle in

life. You taught me well Brenda, and I will use all that you gave me to make us both proud. Your living was not in vain and your legacy will live on through me. I LOVE YOU and thank you for LOVING ME!

Missing you,
Riss

28. BONJOUR *(9/22/10)*

My trip to Paris and Rome was everything I'd hoped it would be! I was completely out of character and couldn't have been happier! I still can't believe that I traveled abroad by myself! I now believe that every woman should travel abroad alone at least once. The independence and confidence it gives you is incomparable. I explored the Paris Metro system, walked more than my body had ever experienced in my life, and participated in back to back bike tours riding through the streets of Paris when I hadn't even looked at a bike since I was in high school. I ate French and Italian food until I was stuffed and drank lots and lots of wine to my heart's content. I can still taste the crepes, pastries, pasta, pizza, and gelato! My heart still skips a beat when I think about how great and cheap the wine was! And for those of you who are unsure, I'm now convinced that Starbucks is everywhere!!

I saw awe-inspiring sights like the Eiffel Tower and The Coliseum. I met Mona Lisa at the Louvre and saw Monet's Beautiful Water Lilies at Musee De L'Orangerie. I saw majestic churches like Notre Dame, Sacre Couer, St Peter's Basilica, and although they wouldn't let us take pictures, Michelangelo's work in the Sistine Chapel is breathtaking and permanently etched in my memory. It's so detailed and grand that you're advised to bring a mirror so that you don't get a nosebleed from looking up so much! I visited my friends Louis Vuitton, and Kenzo and gladly gave them my money! The shopping was absolutely amazing! I felt like the ultimate diva! Not to mention that I did all of this with the little bit of French still in me from High School, my travel books, Brenda's strength and the grace of God. Even better was the confirmation I received on the other side of the Atlantic Ocean that Brenda is indeed with me! I felt her presence so strongly and it's a feeling I will never forget.

I felt it the most when I went to the top of the Eiffel Tower and decided to have dinner on the first level. I made a reservation online to go to the top and felt like a VIP as I whisked past the ridiculously long line. Once at the top, the view of Paris was spectacular! I was so excited and wanted to share the experience with someone yet everyone around me was speaking French. Then out of the blue, I heard English! Without thought, I walked right up to two ladies and started talking a mile a minute! Fortunately, they were friendly! We took a few pictures and shared the moment together. Ironically enough they were visiting from Washington DC so that gave us a little more to talk about.

Upon my decent, I walked in the restaurant 58 Tour Eiffel and with complete confidence, flubbed my French version of "Hello, do you speak English?". The hostess was gracious and we shared a laugh. She then asked if I had a reservation. I didn't but with a little coaxing she squeezed me in. So there I was, having dinner ON the Eiffel Tower! I was so overwhelmed with emotions of joy and sadness. I knew how proud mommy was of me and wished so badly that she was sitting at the table with me in person. I envisioned her being with me when I walked into Kenzo and the staff waited on me hand and foot. I could see her face scrunched up in approval as they draped the new items on her and the subsequent look on her face when they told us how much the items actually cost at the counter! But where else to splurge on oneself and each other than Paris?! Of course we're buying them! I could hear her voice at the Mona Lisa asking if that was what all the fuss was about because truth be told Mona is much smaller than we imagined. Caught up in the moment, I made a champagne toast to her, and as soon as I felt a tear forming, the people at the table next to me struck up a random conversation. I was able to enjoy my 3-course dinner tear free and made some new British friends. All of that...coincidence?? I doubt it!

The trip was a turning point for me. The courage, confidence, and peace I gained are unfathomable. This 5'3 little lady whose only experience "abroad" was going to grandma's house in Jamaica WI traveled alone to a completely foreign country and not only returned to talk about it but had the time of her life! This is the kind of living that Brenda wanted me to do and I know that she's smiling down on me. I came back rejuvenated, ready to move forward knowing that she will always be by my side and will make her presence known when I really need her. Mission Accomplished!

29. I'M GOOD (10/9/10)

It's been a little over six months now since mommy passed away and it's still so hard to believe. Parts of this journey seem just like yesterday. Ironically, on the 6 month anniversary, I had to attend a funeral for a close friend's mother who also passed away from breast cancer and not only attend but sing as requested. This is another time when I knew without the shadow of a doubt that Brenda shows up when I really need her. I was in no condition to sing. The entire experience was overwhelming. My mind kept racing back to the day she left and the aftermath. Seeing my friend's mother's casket from a far because I couldn't bring myself to go to it, and feeling the energy in the room was way too much for me to handle on my own. I just kept repeating to my mom that I needed her and sure enough, I was able to sing the song without making a sniffling fool of myself. I broke down afterwards, but I earned that tear fest.

I can say that at this moment, I'm in a good place. The holidays are fast approaching which will bring another chapter but right now, I'm good. My desire is to keep only positive energy and individuals who share my goal for peace close. I have no desire to go back from whence I came, and had a moment where I was struggling, trying to help others at my own expense, because I had to keep being reminded of that place of darkness and despair that I fought ferociously to get out of. I can't allow anyone or anything to bring me back to that dark place because I'm just getting used to the light again and frankly I'm still vulnerable. This light is different though. Brenda is now a part of that light. She is able to walk with me in spirit to places she could have never gone physically. In that revelation, there is peace. Now instead of picking up the phone, I can just talk out loud and if I listen, I mean really listen, I can hear her. In times of triumph I can hear her say "Go Baby". In times of sorrow and uncontrollable tears I can hear her say, "Come back Riss". Not everyone will understand that but it's not for them to. My walk is mine and mine alone and until I have children, I must live for Brenda and myself. As the old church hymn goes: I've come too far to turn back now.

I've learned so much this year about the people around me. Tragedy truly brings out true colors and I've seen them all. I've forged relationships with people that weren't always close and questioned relationships with those who were and are closest to me. It's par for the course I guess. But I can still say in spite of all of it, that right now, I'm stronger, I'm wiser, I have Brenda in my heart and I'm finally good.

30. TRIGGERS *(11/8/10)*

Something's been brewing for a while now and I can't put my finger on it. While "good", I've been very realistic with the fact that I'm still grieving and that at any moment I could relapse. I'm confident that I won't return to the dark place of previous months but the waves of sadness are becoming more frequent. The upcoming holidays are no help and while trying to stay positive, I am concerned about how I'll handle a new season of "firsts" without my very best friend. The one thing that I've come to terms with is the fact that Brenda was truly the only person who knew me inside and out...and loved me anyway. I told her absolutely everything in confidence knowing that her advice would be objective and free of judgment. If I faltered, I never questioned whether she'd be there to help me dust myself off. If we disagreed, I never worried that she'd no longer be in my corner if I needed her. I've made the painful realization that that relationship was and is the glue that held me together during the hardest of times and I find myself frustrated and pained that I won't have that again in the physical form of her presence.

My mother and I were alike and different in many ways. One of the ways we were alike was her giving spirit. My mother gave her talents, advice, love, encouragement, money and time to a lot of people. Sadly, some of those people didn't deserve it, and while she didn't let that change who she was inherently, those situations hurt her and she never forgot them. I like to call those people parasites. I'm reminded of a previous chapter where I expressed frustration over people talking and not doing. It's not ironic that these parasites were among the number of people I was referring to. I still get irritated when I think about everything my mother did for them and they couldn't even keep their word about coming to visit her in her last days. I know I have to eventually let it go, because they have their own regret to live with but it won't be today.

I've attracted a few of my own over the years and in identifying the parasites this year in particular, it has been a trigger of some of the things my mother went through with ungrateful people and I choose to stop the cycle now. As someone who's already going through the toughest time of my life, I refuse to let anyone else hurt or use me.

I've cleared my heart of anything that was burdening it and left everything on the table with relationships that I've found to be lopsided and superficial. Some relationships have survived and others haven't. However, in each discovery it's just another painful reminder that my friendship with my mother was unmatched. What am I seriously supposed to do for the rest of my life without the one person who I could always turn to? It's my daily struggle. I've noticed an increasing number of evenings where I wake up in the middle of the night sweating profusely. It's actually becoming a nightly event. I don't know if something is going on in my subconscious dreams or if it's a stressor releasing itself, but I do know that some more change is coming in this new chapter.

Yet another trigger, I went to get my baseline mammogram today and that brought a whole new wave of emotion. It was the last thing I wanted to do but I knew it had to be done. I was anxious all weekend about it. When I got to the office I felt myself welling up as I looked around the waiting room. When they called me back into the room for the procedure, I broke down as soon as the tech asked me a simple question. I think she asked me my name. I was reliving everything all over again. I thought about how many times my mother went through this same procedure and let me say, that shit hurt like a hell!! My mind kept racing about how that little painful procedure was just a fraction of everything my mother endured. How she still managed to smile through all the craziness and how she fought to the end.

To no longer have that strength to hold me up through her hurts worse than that damn mammogram. I really miss her so much! I wanted to immediately call her and tell her how I really had no idea of all the pain she went through because of the way she carried her fight. I find myself wondering if I'm really cut out to make it without her because of how important she was to me. I know that I can but in this moment, right now, it's so hard to see it.

31. TIPS FOR THE NON-GRIEVER *(11/28/10)*

I knew it was coming: the sadness, the anger, the bitterness, and the anxiety. I knew that my state of being "good" was temporary. I mean, it *has* been only 8 months and a brand new set of "Firsts" has arrived...The Holidays. This is what perplexes me the most though. Every time I hit the wall, the ones that are supposed to be the closest to me crumble. The ones who promised to always be there and take whatever I dished out because they could never imagine what I'm going through conveniently find a way to dip out until the storm is over.

It's not fair. Perhaps it's my fault for choosing those individuals to play such an important role in my life when they were never ready or equipped to handle the storms of this year. Perhaps, no one can handle these storms that close to me because they are hellacious. But dammit, why?! Am I really supposed to be that strong that only I can help myself through these dark places?? I cry my hardest when I'm alone but am I supposed to? Shouldn't someone get it? One of the biggest purposes of this book was besides being a place for me to vent was to try and help someone to realize that they're not alone in their feelings. But I AM alone in MY feelings.

I was recently told that I was never so needy before. Seriously???? All I could do in that moment was look within and think to myself that I chose this person to be there for me, they had shown their colors before, I looked past it and this is the response I got. Evidently I need to tap into my discernment a little bit more in the future. Are people really that clueless? Again, does not one person GET where I'm at but me? Does it truly take a tragedy in someone's life for him or her to ever get what "being there" means? If so, then that sucks because how are two wounded people supposed to help each other get better? Whenever I have to bring you out of your dark place I'm reminded of my dark places and vice versa. Can you really move forward that way?

Perhaps, but that only seems to drag out the process more with a bunch of emotional setbacks. Why can't Love, Light, Strength, Research and Intuition play a part in defining that role? Unless, those traits were never in the individual to begin with and for that I blame myself and WILL choose better in the future. Do I really need to see a counselor to feel understood again because Brenda was the only person that understood me? How crazy does that sound? I have to PAY someone to get me now! I'm not that fucking complicated!

So now that I've vented, this is where I will help. Here are some tips on how to be there for someone who has lost a close loved one and you in turn have not experienced this tragedy. My delivery may be a little harsh as I'm bitter that I have to break this down, but if you look past the bitterness to the message you won't have to worry about looking like a douche to the person who is going through the toughest time in their life with you being the chosen one to walk beside them.

1. Research- In this day and age of the Internet, there are plentiful resources on grieving. Read a book on grieving, go online and pull up some articles on grieving. Talk to the griever's close friends and family, not just when a situation arises, but regularly. They were there before you and know the griever in a way that will help you cope and know what to do, not do, say and not say.

2. Love- If you ever thought you loved this person, love harder. Whatever was "enough" prior to the day of change for that person will not be enough now. Love harder, Pray harder, Do more and Be harder. In being harder, you need to develop thick skin quickly remembering that what the griever is dishing out to you in anger or sadness still doesn't compare to what they're feeling inside. Take it and leave your ego at the door. When love is involved, the griever will apologize if they went over board or if the anger was misdirected. In your research you will find that everything the griever is feeling is normal and it will be easier to Love them through it when you know it's not you but the process.

3. Light- Be the spark in the griever's day. Keep pettiness, and irrelevant drama out of the equation. You should be the one to make the griever laugh and smile when no one else can. Bring up funny stories from the past. Make

the silly face or statement that only you can make to crack a smile. If you knew the lost loved one, talk about the good times. Keep positivity in the room at all times. Be the light. Just don't be stupid and do stupid things to dim the light.

4. Intuition- Open your heart and mind to try and empathize with where the griever is at in their walk. If we try, all of us have a sixth sense where we can pick up on someone's energy, or the energy in a room, whether it be positive or negative. Adapt to that energy. The only way to adapt to that energy is to remain positive. Positivity will balance positivity and it will always outshine and abolish negativity.

5. Strength- All of the aforementioned tips require strength. These tips are not for runners, quitters, losers, lames, lazy, weak-minded, needy, faint of heart individuals. If you find yourself in any of those categories then you're better off letting the griever know that you're not the person who can be there in that capacity in the days ahead. The truth hurts, but it's easier to let it out in the beginning, than to face the upcoming days, and months when you can't handle it. No one wins in that circumstance, and you won't even make it past a couple of months, because you will have surely bailed feeling beat up and leaving the griever feeling abandoned. The griever will heal quicker without you.

Now if you're wondering "what do I get out of this", then
you REALLY shouldn't be the designated "be there"
person. But if you must know, you will help the griever
get through their walk quicker without unnecessary
emotional set backs caused by you. Which will in turn get
you both to a place of a healthy new normalcy. You'll have
the assurance that when and if the tables are turned and
you have to face a tragedy, that individual will be your
designated "be there" person and will be fully equipped to
help you through your walk because not only have they
been there but they are now healed and will remember
everything you did for them to hold them up. And finally,
you will become a stronger, and better person with a lot of
good karma to redeem. Class dismissed!

32. WE'LL ALWAYS HAVE MUSIC *(11/30/10)*

One of the fondest memories I have of my mother is her love of music. I was raised an "old soul" in this regard. I have so many happy memories with my mom and music. I remember hearing and knowing the entire Rapture album by Anita Baker as a little girl. It was always playing in the car. I saw a tribute to her tonight and it immediately took me back to that "safe place", when mommy was here and we'd both be singing along full blast to her music. It also brought tears, but these were good tears of good memories. I could envision my mother in the room with me saying, "You better saaannnggg girl" and swiping her hand at the TV in approval. I could smile through these tears and I haven't done that in a long time.

Anita was the first soloist I heard that let me know I could sing. Her strong Alto resonated with mine and although she could always hit a note or two that I couldn't quite hit at that age, I'll always remember that it was mommy that introduced her to me. And I'll always remember that she and my dad were my biggest fans. I can hear her now saying, "That's my baby" or "Sannnngggg Riss" with her face scrunched up at any solo or performance I had.

Patti Labelle was another one of mom's favorites. Although I could only sing half the song with Patti because her high soprano would always go off and make me want to sit down somewhere, I remember it fondly. I embrace it and I'll never let it go. My mother had a beautiful voice and she blessed many people with it. In the midst of my tears, heartache, and turmoil, I can still hear it. I know more oldies than someone my age should know but I'm so grateful that she deposited that along with so many other treasures into my life and memory. It's just one more thing to hold on to. And now I know by default that in the midst of tears I can smile. I truly miss you Brenda.

33. CAN SHE HEAR ME? *(12/8/10)*

I sat in my room on my bed last night and had a one sided conversation with my mother. I've spoken out to her before but never like this. This was a snot flying, tears pouring, scream fest that I needed to get out. I simply started out by telling her that I needed her more now than ever before in life and everything else "flowed" from there. I won't reveal the details of my one-sided conversation but I will say that I really just wanted to know if she could hear me.

A lot came out through my tears, sniffles, and shortness of breath. For starters, I can't believe that I'm approaching the nine-month anniversary of her being gone. Three months from a year. This time of year brings a different pain as well separate from the holidays. I realized today that I'm a little less than a month away from the year anniversary of the day that changed my life forever...January 5th at 1:30pm. I will never forget that day. That was the day and time I got the call that my mother's breast cancer had spread to her brain. I had literally just got home from a trip to Miami for New Year's when I got the call. Just like that, I was in my car driving to Albany NY to be with her. It was on the next day that the doctor told me and me only that she had 3-6 months to live and we all know how the timeline decreased from there.

What really shook me to the core today was the fact that I genuinely had NO idea prior to January 6th when the doctor told me mommy's prognosis that she wouldn't survive her fight with cancer. I honestly thought with every fiber of my being that she would be here until I was old and gray. I mean, her mother is still living and her grandmother lived to be up in years before passing away. It just never occurred to me that she would be leaving me so soon in 2010 and would never see me get married or be able to nag me about when I was going to give her some grandbabies. She always knew that I was going to make an impact on this world and when I do kick the door down, she won't be here to see it.

As I mentioned, I had just come home from celebrating New Year's and was so hopeful for all that 2010 had in store for her and I. I would finally land my dream job after being laid off in May of 2009. Mommy would get better and we could get on with living our lives normally without worrying about chemo, radiation treatments, surgeries, etc. Not even a week into the New Year did all those hopes and dreams come crashing down...not even a week.

I often reflect back to January 4th and the days leading up to that fateful call. I was a different woman with different priorities worrying about dumb stuff that I had no control over. Some days I miss the woman I used to be but I recognize at the same time that she couldn't survive the aftermath of this year as she was. That being said, it's difficult to approach this New Year with the same vigor and excitement of years past. Brenda was always the first person I called once the clock struck midnight. I won't be able to do that anymore...ever. It's hard to be hopeful when I can look back to a year ago and see how quickly my desires for the New Year went down the drain within a week's time. I hadn't even really put the New Year on right at that point. I was still getting adjusted to the fit of it when everything I knew changed forever.

As I sit here typing with puffy eyes, I feel a little better that I got it out of my system. I'm going to keep talking out loud to Brenda until I can get to a tear free place. I got caught off guard this time with all my revelations and I'm sure there are more to come. Now, I'm just looking for confirmation that she actually heard me. Stay tuned...

34. IT'S THEIR ANNIVERSARY *(12/18/10)*

On December 18, 1976 my parents began what would be a 33 year marriage in Manhattan NY. They were young, full of hope and dreams of their long and bright new future together. Today would have been their 34th Anniversary. That being said, my thoughts are with my father today. I spoke to him earlier and he told me that although it's a melancholy day he was trying to keep his thoughts on the good times. While saddened, this is a part of his journey that I don't get to walk with him because this was their day together for 33 years. We've been grieving for the same person for some of the same and some very different reasons this year simply because of the various roles my mother played in our lives. Today I have a better understanding of that and I respect it.

In one of our talks my father told me something that at the time I didn't want to hear. He told me that while my mother was special to a lot of people, when she passed away, there were about 5 people whose daily lives were genuinely affected by the aftermath. That I had to understand that after the funeral and memorial service, the majority of the attendees of those services would go back to some sense of normalcy the next day. I found myself resenting those individuals because it seemed so easy for them to get back to their lives and here I stood changed forever. He let me know that as difficult as it was going to be I couldn't live my life like that. And he was right.

Today I focus on the lessons my parents taught me through their marriage and their love for each other in order to pull the positivity out of another milestone without Brenda. I have Christmas and New Year's Eve left before I can close the chapter on the craziest year of my life. For me to say that is an indicator that she has to be with us. I'll focus on that today as well.

35. THIS CHRISTMAS *(12/25/10)*

I'm back in Georgia for a quick trip to spend the holidays
with Aunteee and Unc. I also needed to visit my mother's
site one last time for the year. All the things that we
wanted to do for her site since my last visit in July have
been accomplished. She now has a bench and I even found
some Crosses that are solar powered so her site is lit at
night. In spite of the circumstances it looks good and I'm
happy with the results.

Since Thanksgiving my schedule has been non-stop with
work so I've been in a decent place emotionally out of
necessity. I've had some Scrooge Moments but for the
most part I've been okay. Christmas was usually non-
traditional with our family because my father or I would
be in Jamaica WI visiting my grandmother. Last year,
mommy came down here so it seemed fitting to stand in
her place. That being said, while saddened, I didn't
experience the same anxiety with Thanksgiving because
we weren't normally together this time of year. However,
there was still the missing phone call with her excited
voice on the other line thankful for her gift.

It was really good for me to come down to Georgia and
slow down for a couple of days. I flew in last night and
leave tomorrow night. There's so much family down here
that they keep me busy with joyful distractions. They give
the best hugs too! Last night we went straight from the
airport to a family gathering playing spades, and eating,

coupled with a midnight scripture reading and a hymn. Today was quiet and somber. We had an early dinner full of laughs and memories and afterwards I went to visit mom.

It ironically started to rain when I got on the road, which was symbolic for me. Completely aloof, I drove about 10 minutes out of the way because I missed my turn. Upon my arrival, I talked to her and gave her some messages from loved ones who asked that I deliver them. I cried, but after I got myself together, I walked around the cemetery to see the other stories that surrounded her. I realized today that her site is in between two individuals who passed on in their 50's as well. I also saw a couple of sites of individuals who were taken at a young age. It was humbling to see these other lives represented and to see the same care and love put into their sites by the loved ones left behind. It oddly gave me comfort that I'm not alone in my grieving at this time of year. Mommy's was the most recent passing in that part of the cemetery but they had all been within five years. I knew that like the other individuals that had loved ones laid to rest there, I'd be living a different holiday forever, but that time would continue, and so would I, as they had. As I stood there alone today I knew that I wasn't. There was an unspoken camaraderie that was shared before I had ever gotten there.

I came home drained and slept for about three hours. Tonight I went to an annual Christmas party that one of my cousins puts on every year and had a good time laughing, joking and dancing with family. This Christmas was the first without Brenda but like so many other times in this year I learned something. I learned to look outside the box that I've been in. By doing that I know that I am one of many with a similar story this time of year and every holiday for the rest of our lives. They're making it. And so will I. And so will those who have yet to know our bond.

36. I BID YOU ADIEU *(1/3/11)*

I had to let it really set in that it's a new year before I
wrote this. I have to take a moment and thank God, my
family, friends, loved ones, and strangers, who helped me
get through last year. To be able to sit here and look back
over my journey thus far is unreal. To be able to say that
I'm still standing is a testimony in and of itself. I'm truly
humbled at the Grace that I have received in spite of
myself.

I received so much from 2010. Some of it I will take with
me. Most of it, I will gladly leave behind. I've grown by
leaps and bounds and even though I kicked and screamed
the entire way I can look back to a year ago today and see
a different woman who although not ready, needed to
make her transformation and move closer to her purpose.
I can understand now that every single thing that I
experienced, good, bad and ugly, was necessary. I've been
stretched, bent, cracked, scratched, dropped, burned, and
chipped, but I didn't break. I have a conviction beyond
anything I ever believed before that in spite of the
hardest year of my life, I'm still blessed. I'm blessed with a
spirit that resides within me and took me through the
fire. That spirit is Brenda. I can't hear her voice, see her
face, or hug her but I know she's with me protecting me
and guiding me. There is no way that I would be here
right now if it wasn't true. I understand now why I had to
cry my hardest by myself. I would have never blossomed

into that Lotus that sits on top of the dark and murky water if I didn't. I can gladly sit atop of that darkness victorious. I just now, had the revelation that Brenda was already a Lotus here on earth. She had to go on so that I could become a Lotus too. All this time I thought that she became the Lotus in passing but that's furthest from the truth. She endured her darkness and rose above it a long time ago. I see it now Brenda and I thank you.

I kept pushing back writing this chapter because I knew I would be emotional. I'm just so overwhelmed at all that I've overcome. I honestly had no idea how I was going to make it to this day and this year. The grief and despair would grip me so tightly at times, that I honestly thought that I was losing my mind. It's true that life goes on. Whether you're going to participate in it or not is up to you. I remember that one of the things Brenda said she wanted to be remembered for was being my mother. It was something about the *way* she said it that sticks with me. She said it with a conviction that I will never forget. Like she knew that I was destined for something great. The woman I was a year ago today wasn't prepared for whatever it was going to be, but the woman I present to you today is because, and only because of 2010.

I cursed 2010 even up to today. I was so ready to get the hell out of that awful year full of loss, sadness, and fear. But if it hadn't been for 2010, I wouldn't be ready for my next step. Brenda knew that and she always knew I was going to make it even when I couldn't see it. The woman I was a year ago wouldn't have dreamed of traveling to Paris by herself. The woman I was a year ago was settling for a life that wouldn't have allowed her to reach her full potential. The woman I am today has a fire within that would have burned the hell out of the woman I was a year ago. I'm only moving forward and I gladly bid the woman I was a year ago "adieu".

37. BREAKING PLATES TO TD JAKES *(1/8/11)*

This week was hazy for me. I was always a step behind and simply a little "off" from my normal self. The conviction and confidence from my last chapter are still there but I still fight with the sadness and anger. As I've stated in previous chapters, January 5th and 6th marked the one-year anniversary of the beginning of my journey and the last days I would have with my mother. On the 5th, we found out that mommy's breast cancer spread to her brain. On the 6th the doctor told me that it was in fact terminal. It's still numbing.

I went through my usual waves of sadness to anger to new normalcy. Wednesday was my sad day. Thursday was my angry day. Friday I found some additional peace. On Wednesday, I immediately woke up sad. I was busy with errands and projects to keep me occupied and a couple of my friends sent me messages letting me know that they were thinking of me, which always helps. Thursday night in particular was interesting because my anger had hit a high point. Sometimes I find myself so wrapped up in the bitterness of feeling alone and the unfairness of my mother not being here anymore that I become enraged. In this place, I begin to focus on the negative parts of my journey, like the key individuals who never understood how to be there for me (and still don't), instead of focusing on the ones who shined and were consistent in showing me love and support. I know that I should focus on the fact that I was strong enough to let those people go, but when I'm hurting my mind can't help but go there.

In the midst of my anger, I tried one of my new coping mechanisms...breaking plates! When my family came to visit me for Thanksgiving, I expressed this new coping mechanism to my aunteee. A random fact about me, that I'm not proud of, is that I sometimes break valuable things (i.e. my phone) in a fit of rage. God is still working on me! I decided that instead, I would break things that weren't valuable like dishes, in my backyard, to release my anger. Aunteee thought it was a good idea and rearranged my dishes so that the mismatched plates would be the ones I could break. Once I got through those, I could go to the Dollar store and buy some cheap ones. Now this coping mechanism was just a theory and I hadn't done it...until Thursday. I have to say, that while it felt absolutely amazing in the moment, it was only a short-term fix. I still needed to address the source of my anger.

Cue in Friday. One of my new acquaintances let me know about a revival that her church was having and that TD Jakes was going to preach. During this process, although I've never turned my back on my faith and my Christian beliefs, lets just say that my relationship with God has been a little strained. I truthfully hadn't been to church since April or May. At the time I was finding myself completely overwhelmed with emotions every time I went and it was too much for me to handle. In turn, I began convincing myself not to go because I was tired amongst other excuses until I just stopped going all together. So when asked to go the revival, needless to say, I was less than thrilled. However, my spirit told me to say yes. As soon as I said yes, I started to change my mind because I was genuinely tired on Friday from work and just wanted to sit in the house. The excuses were coming a mile a minute. That's when I stopped myself and forced myself to go because I knew that something was trying to keep me from my blessing. I made the best decision of my early 2011 with that choice. The service and sermon were wonderful, I cried like a baby and I began to address the source of my anger, which is a much more effective and long-term solution.

I realized in my strained relationship with God that I was upset because I felt that God took my mother from me when I wasn't ready. Last night I remembered that she had given a great fight, was tired, and in turn ready to leave so He gave her rest. I realized that my mother equipped me with all the tools to be able to make it without her. She had been planting seeds of wisdom and love in my life throughout my life and they only needed to be watered. My tears watered them and they're growing within me now. I am a living embodiment of all of the good my mother was. I see her looking back at me in the mirror more and more everyday. My anger was blocking my view and I readily released it on Friday at the service. It could have been very easy for me to learn how to live in my anger while continuing to break dishes, but she and

He desire so much more for me. I'm still growing and learning, and will still have to fight the waves of anger and sadness that come at me. However, I'm finally addressing the source of the issue. Now when I smile at myself in the mirror, I see Brenda smiling back at me...and we look good!

38. PINK ROSES *(1/18/11)*

I debated if I would share this experience but I have to be fearless. I've started something here and if it's going to continue to help others and myself I have to be honest. So, with that being said, I talked to a psychic today on the phone or as I like to put it so I don't sound so crazy "a lady with a special gift of clairvoyance". I spoke to one in the early part of 2010 while my mother was still here and while she had some interesting points that proved true, when she started talking about how I was persecuted in my past lives I got a little weirded out!

However, since losing mom, it had been on my mind and heart and I waited for the right confirmation to talk to a new one. It's okay if you call me crazy but I do believe that there are people on this earth that have special gifts of foresight. While my mother didn't have people paying to speak with her, she had discernment when it came to me, and those around me. If I was ever losing focus in college she would call and simply ask me "What are you doing?". Her tone, never scolding would put me back on track with my studies. By my Junior year she reluctantly gave me room to make my own mistakes but whenever my mother warned me about someone I was hanging out with, it was never long after that her warning would ring true.

In a recent conversation with one of my girlfriends who is also a Christian, she brought up speaking to one and I knew that was my sign to check her out. It was definitely interesting. She did indeed have some insight and she touched on some points that she couldn't have known on her own. She noted a loss in my life. I told her my mother and she then asked if it was cancer. Whoa #1. She then said she was seeing a soft pink rose. Whoa #2.

Pink was my mother's favorite color and we have a special story about roses. When I was younger, whenever I introduced my mother to a guy I was dating (which wasn't often), she would go into her "Perfect Rose" speech. How her daughter was a perfect rose and while he was dating her daughter not one petal should fall off. Man, I can't wait to do that to my unborn daughter! I actually have a rose as one of the charms on the charm bracelet I bought last year. Every charm is a reminder of my mother and the rose represents this story.

The conversation with "the lady with the special gift of clairvoyance" continued and she told me that my mother is no longer suffering, is with me, wants me to enjoy life and if I want to talk to her, all I have to do is speak out loud because she can hear me. Sounds familiar right? I started to believe that I'm actually psychic because she was telling me stuff that I already believed, but unsure I still needed confirmation. She got into some other stuff that got a little "side eye" from me, but I got off the phone feeling better than I did when I called, so it served its purpose. Will I call back? I have no clue. But I'm glad I did this time.

I put this out there because while unorthodox, it was a necessary step for me. I needed to make that call. Even if the lady wound up being completely crazy with no gift whatsoever at least I know I tried. She only confirmed in my spirit what I already believed. If that's crazy then so be it but I'm one step further on this path and the answers are coming. Slowly but surely, they are coming and I'm ready for them.

39. STRENGTH IN NUMBERS *(1/25/11)*

It's hard to believe that it's been 10 months since March 24th. It's even harder to believe that there are only two months left to close this chapter. I've come to consider this year the first chapter of my new life. Countless individuals have told me that the first year is the most difficult in the grieving process. It's not to assume that after the first year, life goes back to normal but the "firsts" after a great loss are by far the most challenging.

My emotions while stable as compared to previous months still have the room to fluctuate. However the tears that come now mostly stem from a more positive place. I realize a little bit more everyday how much Brenda loved and cherished me. I well up with emotion in those moments because I am blessed to know that love. I see now that without my knowledge at the time, my mother was constantly putting parameters in place that would ensure I wanted for nothing mentally, emotionally, and financially when she left in the physical form. Seeing that now, while I still miss her and want nothing more than to have her here with me, I almost feel fortunate because she gave me what so many other people aren't as lucky to receive...she prepared me for her departure.

As a result, lately I've been looking outside of myself more and paying attention to others' circumstances. It was not easy at all for me to step out of my pity party and begin to look outward. I'm certain a lot of people who are grieving don't even get to this place because the pain of the loss is so deep and hurts so badly, it's virtually impossible to look outside of oneself.

I believe that this process is necessary because it's your defense mechanism kicking in and protecting you from any additional hurt. Anything that doesn't deal with the healing from your loss becomes irrelevant. In the midst of my grief, I found myself very apathetic to surrounding drama. I'm certain that it made me appear to be very cold and jaded at the time but essentially I was. Friends that would normally come to me to get advice or a listening ear learned quickly that the "new me" didn't have the energy or desire to provide either. In self-preservation mode, your spirit will only allow you to deal with so much before it shuts down so that you can focus on healing the major wound and void at hand.

It's a survival technique. However, without the proper tools, it's very easy to stay in this place and in the long term it becomes unhealthy. I'm grateful that I was given the tools to cope from Brenda. But this brings me back to my original point. What do you do if you weren't given the gift of preparation? How do you cope then? This is where I find my mind going as I think about the individuals who woke up today believing they'd see their loved one again after work or school and got the call that we all dread. What do they do? How can I help?

Now that I'm slowly approaching the stage of (dare I say it) acceptance, I'm finally able to look outside of my loss and see that not only are there other people hurting but their hurt is more recent than mine. It brings me to tears because I remember the despair. I remember the apathy. I remember truly believing that I would never stop crying and screaming. I remember believing that I would never make it out of that dark place.

 A major reason that I've come as far as I have is because of the preparation I was given. While I wasn't prepared for the moment of losing Brenda because no matter how hard you try, you're never prepared for that moment. I was prepared for the aftermath, unbeknownst to me at the time. For that I'm grateful and for that I must help someone else who's hurting.

After three months of going back and forth trying to set up a meeting with an acquaintance who had recently lost her mother to cancer, we finally sat down to talk. We didn't really know much about each other beyond surface conversations but we learned that we shared a lot in common. As much as she says I helped her, she has no idea how much she helped me. In this stage of what I'll call "Pre-Acceptance", there's a peace in knowing that I'm not alone in my thoughts and feelings from someone who is still in it like I am. While I wouldn't wish what I feel and have felt on my worst enemy, I believe that there's a reason our paths finally crossed. Every time I told her that what she was feeling wasn't crazy, it was a confirmation for me that I'm not crazy either! Although through my research, I knew that I wasn't, there's always strength in numbers to help prove a theory. I left our meeting feeling great and with the knowledge that everything I went through wasn't in vain if I use my experience to help someone else. That's exactly what Brenda would have done, and being her daughter I have no choice but to follow suit. It took some time for me to get here but there's no place I'd rather be.

40. WHO'S THAT GIRL? *(1/30/11)*

Although this walk has had the lowest points of my life, I find myself acknowledging the highs more and more lately. I have grown more in this span of a little more than ten months than I have for most of my life when Brenda was still here. There's an irony in that realization that I'm still wrapping my head around. It feels like right before she left she sprinkled some Miracle Grow on me and I've been growing by leaps and bounds ever since.

Being the spoiled only child that I am, I actually used to wait for my mother to come to town every couple of months and help me organize and clean my house (and by help me, I mean she did it all by herself). My friends are amazed when they see my house now and even more amazed that I keep it up on my own (not as good as Brenda though). The same girl, who never made her bed for days on end before, can't start her day without making it first. The same girl who used to squander all of her money away actually has a savings account now and those are just the little, everyday things.

I honestly believe that I lost my mind in a good way with this newfound adventurous spirit. I still look at my pictures from Paris and Rome in disbelief that I picked up and traveled abroad all by myself. And when I got over there, had the nerve to master public transportation, and go on bike tours in the middle of the busy Paris streets and intersections. This self-proclaimed Diva with awful allergies has gone zip lining in the woods at heights of 2-3 story homes above the ground without a safety net. Yes...Me!

I can now add Skiing and Snow Tubing to my list of accomplishments. Now this idea wasn't initiated by me but once presented, I surprisingly agreed to it. A year ago and in previous years, you wouldn't catch me on anyone's slope. I grew up in Rochester NY and went to college in New Hampshire. Clearly if I hadn't tried it in all those years, it wasn't on my bucket list of things to do but again, I'm not just living for myself anymore. I'm living for Brenda too and I promised that I would do all the things she never had the chance to. So that's the attitude I took. That being said, I actually enjoyed myself! Snow tubing was much more fun and much less work but once I stopped falling (and I fell a lot), skiing grew on me. I am sore beyond belief at this moment but I am so proud of myself for trying and I know that she is too!

I believe another turning point for me in this journey has been embracing what Brenda wanted for me. She genuinely wanted me to be happy and to live life to the fullest. It would be disappointing to her to have placed all these resources at my feet and I let them all go to the wayside because I was consumed with my grief and anger. It took her leaving for me to find the inner strength to do all of these things but had she not placed it in me to begin with, I wouldn't be doing them with or without her here and I get that now too. I feel so fortunate to have been blessed with her for the time I had her. As much as I loved and adored her while she was here, my love has grown for her even more and that's what keeps me going...and I will keep going. I love you so much Brenda, and WE have a lot more life to live!

41. I REMINISCE *(2/18/11)*

In this newfound normalcy, it's very easy for me to get caught up in life. My career keeps me busy and usually before I know it, another week has passed. I've created a routine and have begun to function well in it. I think of Brenda often but I don't really get that sad anymore (waves come and go), as I've been really trying to embrace the lessons and epiphanies I've had as of late. However, every once in a while I get a reminder that as much as I have fooled myself into thinking that all is well, she's not going to be there if I pick up the phone to call her.

Today at work (I'm in sales), our territories were realigned and as representatives we weren't given any foresight to how major the changes were going to be. I lost some accounts that were important to me but in return because of my performance over the last year, I received some very prestigious accounts that I never intended or believed would be mine. A major thing I learned about myself over this last year is my disdain for change, specifically when it's not by my hand. My life has been jostled so much for obvious reasons that unexpected change gives me anxiety. I found myself stressed out in the office after my division manager informed me of the "good news". He was talking and I was nodding my head yes, giving my best poker face, but my mind was racing, and I felt tightness in my chest. At the time I couldn't put my finger on why I was feeling the way I was. I talked with my boyfriend about it and while he did a great job encouraging me I still felt unsettled. It was upon coming home from dinner that it hit me that a major link in my chain of events was missing.

A year ago, I would have received the news of my new territory, and while happy yet unsure, I would have called Brenda as soon as I left the building to freak out on the phone. She would calm me the hell down and tell me that I was tripping. That I was given a great opportunity, and that I was going to exceed above and beyond my or their expectations. In typical Brenda fashion, she would have ended the conversation with a "Go Baby". As I'm typing this, I'm smiling and tearing up reminiscing on this same conversation that we had hundreds of times in reference to different circumstances in my life (man, I miss her). At the same time, remembering this conversation gives me the confirmation that I'm going to knock it out the box with my new responsibilities. She was my number one fan and always reminded me of who I was and whose I was. I sometimes forget now that she's not here. Now that I've placed the root of my anxiety I feel better. Not because I can change the cause, but because once pinpointed, I can find my way out of it.

42. 24 *(3/1/11)*

Less than a month from a year and I can honestly say that I don't know what or how to feel about it. I've thrown myself into my career as a means to not have too much time to think or get sad. Staying busy is my therapy as of late. I don't want to think about it because I don't know where it will take me in the moment. The last 24 days of mommy's life in particular are extremely vivid to me. I can't look back over any series of days in my life from a previous year with the same detail in my memories. A year ago on Monday morning I sent my parents off to Georgia. I remember all the emotions I felt. The confusion, the fear, the sadness, and the uncertainty all come rushing back to me in moments of silence. I remember mommy's face and demeanor. I remember how tired she looked. She knew that on that trip to Georgia she wasn't coming back to Albany. She knew she was headed to her resting place but she just had to hold on a little while longer.

I remember feeling so empty and drained after they left, because deep down in my heart I knew what mommy knew, but unlike her I wasn't ready to receive it. As much as I had pumped myself up that I could let her go so she could rest, I knew that I was serving myself a nice big heaping plate of BS. These upcoming days are the most vivid because I knew the end was coming. I could hear it in her voice everyday on the phone as her condition declined. At this point a year ago, I knew that she wasn't going to get better. I knew that it was a matter of time before my life would never be the same again. It's weird to see it a year later because now I know the precise day and hour that my life changed. Then, I was still hoping that maybe she could make it to another Mother's Day, or my birthday in June. When it all came crashing down, I can look back to a year ago today and say that I honestly had no clue what was in store for me or that I would have less than 24 days left with my mother here on earth.

I know I made the best of it, but I still look back and wish there were things I had done better. I wish I videotaped her more. I wish I asked her more questions while she could still talk. I wish I had been better prepared for her pain management with the new doctor in Georgia at the end because that was her main wish in her living will. It all happened so much sooner than I thought it would or should have. I wish most of all that I knew then that I only had 24 days left.

The emotions I bottle up always come out when I write. I'll go through my everyday motions without acknowledging what's going on inside, but I always release it here whether I want to or not. I still miss her, I still cry hard and I still struggle. In these moments it doesn't feel easier at all.

43. THE FINAL STRETCH *(3/21/11)*

I have literally done everything possible to delay writing
this chapter because of the unknown of where it will take
me emotionally tonight. A year ago I was in the hospital
with mommy...confused, fearful, sad, and angry. This has
been the busiest month I've had in a long time and for
good reason. Idle time is not my friend so I avoid it at all
costs. During the week, I run myself ragged with work,
and on the weekend I go out of town. I visited my
grandmother in Jamaica this month and found myself in
a different place than I was when I went last year. Last
year, I was fresh off of losing mom and needed to get
away. I was perfectly fine with going to the beach during
the day and staying in the house at night. I didn't go out
at all. I simply read books and slept. This year I thought I
would have the same experience but not so much. After
two nights in the house, I had to get out and found myself
at the resort down the road to occupy my time and mind
in the evenings. My mind will race a mile a minute if I let
it but as of right now, I'm in control of it.

I dragged all morning as my own personal protest to
beginning this week because this is THE week. The one-
year anniversary of my mother's cross over is
approaching quicker than I could have ever imagined.
Has it really been almost a year since she left me? Has it
really been almost a year in this new normalcy? Am I
really still standing, functioning, thriving and moving
forward without her here? This moment a calendar year

ago, I was in the hospital with her literally freaking out. I was drained but alert at the same time listening for her breaths. I clearly remember every moment. Going into the hospital believing that I had more time with her than I really did. Shocked to find out that I was completely mistaken and even the doctor's prediction of how much longer she would be here was wrong. I left the hospital riding with her in an ambulance believing I had two weeks. By the time we got her to aunteee's house, the hospice nurse said 2-3 days, and she was gone before daylight came again. 55 years gone in the blink of an eye and I'm left with the responsibility to share the lessons without the teacher.

She still hasn't come to me in dreams like I thought she would but I'm going to remain faithful that she's only going to come when I really need her. For her to think that I haven't really needed her over this past year is crazy to me but I interpret it as her way of saying that I'm doing okay on my own. I had no strategy on how to get through this week besides getting through it as fast as I could by staying busy, but my dad suggested that we meet in Georgia where mom is laid to rest on the day of her passing. I have mixed emotions as this is the complete antithesis of how I wanted to handle the anniversary but it will probably be for the best as we'll be together as a family. I've had questions answered, epiphanies, breakdowns and breakthroughs along this journey but this is the first time where I genuinely don't know what or how to feel. I'm simply numb.

44. BRENDA TAUGHT ME *(3/25/11)*

The last two days have been trying to say the least but somehow I made it. I woke up very heavy on Wednesday morning because it was Wednesday morning when mom passed last year. In an attempt to boost my spirits I went to get my hair done and broke down into tears at the first inquiry of my sad countenance. I pulled it together and left the salon feeling a little better. I attempted to go to Georgia that evening for a quick less than 24-hour trip in order to visit mom's site with my dad and that's when the craziness started.

I got on the plane that was on time for 6:45 and promptly fell asleep for an hour to only wake up and find us still sitting on the tarmac in Baltimore due to inclement weather. Another hour passes and someone on the plane has a medical emergency so we have to go back to the gate for them to tell us that even after they remove the ill passenger, it could be another 40 minutes before we're in the air. At this point it's 9pm and my return flight was at 1:45 the next day as I had an important meeting for work. Keep in mind that once I actually got to Atlanta, there was still an hour and a half drive to get to Warner Robins. So needless to say, I elected to get off the plane... with my bag still checked on the plane heading to Atlanta. Feeling sorry for myself I went to grab some food and had a few libations to take the edge off. I managed to stay awake until 3:30am, which was the actual time of her passing thanks to one of my girlfriends who came out to keep me company and promptly took my drunken self to bed afterwards.

Cue in Thursday, I woke up miserable and laid in bed until 12:30 when I finally forced myself to get up. I had some running around to do for work before my five-hour meeting beginning at 5pm. I literally ran around like a crazy lady until the meeting and was occupied for the rest of the evening. After the meeting I came home talked to my dad, commenced a good, hearty tear fest and went to bed without any major fanfare.

So all in all, I got through it. I've commemorated other milestones in the past year but this one in particular was very different. I didn't want to commemorate the day Brenda left me. I didn't want to celebrate, acknowledge or re-live the day that I lost my best friend and my life changed forever. There was no action that seemed appropriate besides getting through the day.

So where does that leave me now? I'm now officially on the other side of a year without Brenda and today I'm okay. I'm definitely better than I was yesterday and a part of it is because she makes her presence known more now. She still guides me, and warns me of potential dangers. She still gives me signs to help me move in the right direction. There are countless instances where I'll be on the verge of forgetting something and I'll get a unique reminder i.e. my keys drop, or my phone rings before I walk out the door to leave it. While these could be coincidence, I truly believe differently. I have to believe differently.

A year ago today, I was completely lost. The despair was so bad in the first couple of days that I actually slept with her wig because that was all I had to feel close to her. For those of you who have never lost a close loved one and find it hard to relate, think on that...I slept with a wig because I wanted her to come back that badly. I'm a far cry from that girl today but it's only because of the Grace of God and what Brenda instilled in me. To this very day, I'm learning and remembering the lessons she taught me. Brenda taught me well and today I remember all of it:

Brenda taught me to love and respect myself SO much that everyone else HAS to follow suit.
Brenda taught me how to elegantly walk in a room.
Brenda taught me to be fearless.
Brenda taught me to be independent and outspoken.
Brenda taught me to never settle.
Brenda taught me who I am and Whose I am.
Brenda taught me how to be compassionate.
Brenda taught me how to be objective.
Brenda taught me how to be a Lady.
Brenda taught me to not be judgmental.
Brenda taught me how to get my point across.
Brenda taught me how to smile in the face of adversity.
Brenda taught me Grace.
Brenda taught me Tact.

Brenda taught me how to lead by example.

Brenda taught me how to give and earn respect.

Brenda taught me how to guard my heart.

Brenda taught me how to "lose weight", weight being unhealthy relationships.

Brenda taught me that it takes a long time to grow an old friend.

Brenda taught me that not everyone will treat me the way I treat them but to never let it change me.

Brenda taught me that I'm Great enough.

Brenda taught me how to give of my time, my talents, my love, and myself.

Brenda taught me that I can do ALL things through Christ who strengthens me.

And so much more...Brenda taught me. I know that lady loved me with every ounce of her being and based on everything Brenda taught me, I must make her proud.

45. A NEW LEASE *(4/12/11)*

I'm on the other side of the year of my new normalcy and in a completely different space mentally, emotionally, and spiritually than I was this time last year for obvious reasons. After a year of struggle, and heartache I remember one of the things my mother wanted the most for me and my life was to be fully, and genuinely happy. I tolerated and accepted a lot of things I didn't deserve last year from various people for various reasons. I can look back now and understand why. I truly desired to keep the snapshot of what my life was before Brenda left the same and sometimes to my detriment. I was so fixated on the idea that mommy only left here because she believed that I was in good hands with the people in my circle at that moment that I didn't pay attention to the fact my hands alone were good enough.

She always knew I would thrive because of what she placed inside of me over the 32 years of my life that I was blessed to share with her. It was never about THEM. It was always about ME. Having that moment of clarity changed me forever and removed a great burden of resentment that I had toward a couple people in my inner circle and truthfully Brenda too. I would get so angry at her in the depths of my grief because I would convince myself that she had to know better. She had been so on point with warning me about those around me in the past. I recall being alone screaming out loud in my room and asking how she could possibly leave me with them. In that mindset it seemed that she was so ready to leave here that she actually convinced herself that they'd help hold me up when deep down she knew differently. Thankfully I know the truth now.

As I grew, people either grew with me or we grew apart. I found myself stunting my growth on several occasions as I desperately tried to keep the relationships that existed in that snapshot of my life pre March 24th 2010. However, messages weren't being received and I remained frustrated. Already because of the fact that the growth I was experiencing was nothing that I initiated or necessarily wanted and then doubly because the process seemed like it was being drawn out. This year had to be different. I know now that mom wouldn't have been happy or tolerated the things I went through had she still been here in the aftermath. For the sake of not being able to talk to her on the phone or in person did it take me a little longer to figure out that I was ultimately no longer on the path to happiness in my everyday life and I needed to make changes ASAP.

So I did. I found the courage to let go of relationships and circumstances that were not healthy or helpful to me. As a result, I have taken back the control that I lost. I lost control of my emotions and am re-training myself on how to deal with the people in my life that are supposed to be here. I spent so much time fussing, cussing, and screaming because I wasn't being heard when I spoke politely, that now I have to remember how to bring it down a few notches. There's no need to yell and justify myself when those who are supposed to be here are listening. They already understand and have either walked with me or walked a similar walk.

I was struggling with anger and bitterness towards myself because of what I allowed myself to go through and towards those who inflicted the unnecessary drama and setbacks. However, I've forgiven myself as well as them. It was all supposed to happen because had I never experienced the negative; I wouldn't appreciate the positive that has come and is coming. I'm so grateful for the lightness I now feel and the smile that has always lived within but got lost in the shuffle. My goal is to never take it for granted. Brenda didn't leave here because she knew those around me were going to hold me up. She left here knowing that I would be able to do it myself...and I did, with the Grace of God, and her strength that flows through my veins, I did and I will. I welcome Love, Joy, Peace, Hope, and Happiness because I know that the storm prepared me for my New Lease on life!

46. EPILOGUE-LOOK AT ME NOW *(2/20/12)*

I wrote the last chapter of this book a little shy of a year ago. I was just beginning to get used to the new skin I found after such a tumultuous year. I was shedding what I believed were the final layers of negativity that plagued me for much of that year. However, I still had a lot of work to do. As I approached acceptance, I still struggled with my grief over Brenda. I would still think of how unfair it was for her to leave me so soon. I would still find myself flustered that I couldn't run to her for quick guidance and instead had to take the much slower route of searching within for the answers. I still struggled with the loss of key relationships in my life as a result of my transformation and my desire to see if those relationships could eventually be reconciled. I still struggled with my expectations of people, especially new people who entered my life. But all of it was necessary.

Looking back over the last year, I know that my acceptance of everything I endured from January 5th 2010 forward didn't truly come until September 2011. I was on a "stay-cation" because truthfully I spent all of the money my mother had initially left for me and I couldn't afford to go on the big trip abroad like I did the year before. My at times excessive retail "therapy" was only a short-term fix for what I was dealing with internally. Once the temporary thrill of a great buy wore off and I was forced to feel my grief, like an addict, I went shopping again. While I did some great things with the money, I did some foolish things as well. I was coerced to realize once the money ran out, that I was never going to be able to run from my grief. I had to face it head on. Let the real healing begin...

In addition, I had sent out about twenty transcripts of the first copy of this book and received rejection letter after rejection letter. My great promotion at work that I spoke of in a previous chapter was not working out the way I planned and put an unexpected and severe pinch on my pockets. And I was going through all of this without my best friend Brenda to give me the boost I needed, as well as the reminder, that as it had always been, I would make it through this funk too.

I was frustrated with myself, full of self-pity and in dire need of inspiration. At my wits end, I went to the newly opened Martin Luther King Jr. Monument in Washington DC on Friday the 16th and I finally found myself in church after a very long hiatus that Sunday. It was in church that I was given the scripture that for the first time put my mother's passing in crystal clear perspective. It was II Timothy 4:7- "I have fought a good fight. I have finished my race. I kept the faith." That was it! Someone could've probably told me that scripture a thousand times before that day but in that moment it clicked. Everything about my mother's battle with breast cancer and depression is in that one little verse. She wasn't "taken" from me. She simply finished her race and in turn passed the baton on to me.

With that being said, I had to ask myself "Why on earth am I standing still"? I had started a Non-Profit Organization in March of 2011 in honor of my mother named LotusFlyy and had yet to do anything outside of getting the state to recognize us. My family had also put together an endowment at her Alma Mater, Roberts Wesleyan College, that when fulfilled would fund a scholarship for Breast Cancer Survivors or the kin of "Sheroes" who passed away from it. My original plan was to have proceeds from this book be my contribution to the endowment and it still is, but after the original version was rejected, I kindly retreated in the corner and did nothing else but nurse my bruised ego. It took so much out of me to edit the book the first time because I had to revisit and relive each chapter. Who would sign up for that again? This crazy girl would, knowing that a part of her purpose is getting this book done. I knew that it was going to take time and I knew that I had to mentally and emotionally prepare myself to walk this path again. I didn't know when or how the opportunity would arise but I did know that in the meantime I had to do something to honor my mother and contribute to her legacy.

In perfect timing, some tough love from a good friend telling me to stop being complacent pushed me forward. With a lot of help from family, friends, and even strangers, we put together a Breast Cancer Awareness Happy Hour as LotusFlyy to raise funds for the endowment in a month's time in late October. The restaurant was filled to capacity and we raised over

$1400 in one night! I took all the negativity that I was still harboring and poured that energy into something very positive. I began to speak positivity in my life everyday knowing that was Brenda's heart for me. Slowly but surely I began to see a shift when I took the energy off of myself and put it into a cause bigger than me. After the happy hour I knew that I had only chipped the iceberg but I also knew that this book still needed to come to fruition or I'd be attempting to do a happy hour every month!

This brings me to my annual trip to Grandma's house in Jamaica, which is where I am right now. I knew that this would be the perfect place to sequester myself and finally finish it. I could go to the beach during the day and lock myself in my room at night giving me an opportunity to truly feel the moments again and release them without having to explain myself or feelings to anyone.

Now I understand why it took so long for me to get to this final stage of editing. My last chapter is full of hope as it should be because that was the space I was in, but it can also lead you to believe that I ran off into the sunset full of acceptance of the loss of my mother never to struggle again. That's furthest from the truth. I didn't want you to have a false expectation of your journey and your grieving process. The truth is that there is no time limit on how long it takes one to reach the point of peace and acceptance. A year was still way too soon for me even though I acknowledge that I was becoming more accepting of acceptance. I still had some kinks to iron out and I still will almost two years later and for years to come.

I'm still a work in progress. I still don't know how I'm going to approach my mother's two-year anniversary but I know that I'll get through it and while not easy it will be a little easier than last year. Isn't that all we can really ask for? It's not realistic to expect all, let alone any, of the pain to go away. But it is realistic to expect that how you approach and handle the pain will improve.

Knowing that my mother finished her race on her terms and passed her legacy on to me gives me something to believe in and work towards. I now have somewhere to focus my energy and redirect the negativity I sometimes feel. I truly pray that sharing my crazy and twisted journey with you helped you find your acceptance or at the very least helped you find the path towards it. Your peace lies above the dark and murky waters that grief left you in and what a beautiful Lotus bloom you will be!

www.ingramcontent.com/pod-product-compliance
Lightning Source LLC
Chambersburg PA
CBHW022114280326
41933CB00007B/387